Exercise Testing and Training in the Elderly Cardiac Patient

Current Issues in Cardiac Rehabilitation
Monograph Number 1

Mark A. Williams, PhD
Creighton University

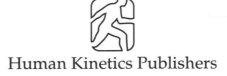

Human Kinetics Publishers

Library of Congress Cataloging-in-Publication Data

Williams, Mark Alan, 1951-
   Exercise testing and training in the elderly cardiac patient /
Mark A. Williams.
       p.   cm. -- (Current issues in cardiac rehabilitation ;
monograph no. 1)
   Includes index.
   ISBN 0-87322-621-6
   1. Heart--Diseases--Exercise therapy.   2. Exercise tests.
3. Exercise for the aged.   4. Aged--Rehabilitation.   I. Title.
II. Series.
RC684.E9W55   1994
618.97'612062--dc20
                                                                93-34283
                                                                CIP

ISBN: 0-87322-621-6

ISSN: 1071-7889

Copyright © 1994 by Mark A. Williams

Developmental Editor: Marni Basic
Assistant Editors: Lisa Sotirelis and John Wentworth
Copyeditor: Jane Bowers
Proofreader: Tom Rice
Indexer: Theresa J. Schaefer
Production Director: Ernie Noa
Typesetting and Layout: Angela K. Snyder, Yvonne Winsor, and Tara Welsch
Cover and Text Design: Keith Blomberg
Illustrations: Keith Blomberg
Printer: United Graphics

Printed in the United States of America

10   9   8   7   6   5   4   3   2   1

Human Kinetics Publishers
Box 5076, Champaign, IL 61825-5076
1-800-747-4457

Canada: Human Kinetics Publishers, Box 24040, Windsor, ON N8Y 4Y9
1-800-465-7301 (in Canada only)

Europe: Human Kinetics Publishers (Europe) Ltd.,
P.O. Box IW14, Leeds LS16 6TR, England
0532-781708

Australia: Human Kinetics Publishers, P.O. Box 80, Kingswood 5062, South Australia
618-374-0433

New Zealand: Human Kinetics Publishers, P.O. Box 105-231, Auckland 1
(09) 309-2259

Dedicated to my wife, Kelly, and my sons, John and Alec

Contents

Preface

How old would you be if you didn't know how old you were?

Leroy "Satchel" Paige

Elderly persons, both with and without cardiovascular disease, make up the fastest growing segment of the U.S. population. But as recently as the mid- to late 1970s, elderly patients were discouraged from participating in exercise training programs after acute myocardial infarction or coronary artery bypass graft surgery, and patients aged 65 or greater were often excluded from these activities. In the early 1980s, my colleagues and I began to question this limitation, primarily because many elderly patients were otherwise eligible for our rehabilitation program and were excited about participating but were excluded simply because of age. At that time we began to systematically study elderly patients' acute responses to exercise following exercise training. In 1985, we published the first report of exercise training in elderly cardiac patients (278).

Since I began working more with elderly patients, I have observed the tremendous potential that most of them possess. In fact, many elderly patients are among our most dedicated participants. They possess an enthusiasm for life that is enviable, and yet they understand their limitations and do all they can to remain active and healthy. I asked one patient, "Is everything all right, Will?" Will, a 78-year-old post–myocardial infarction participant, had just completed exercising at a bicycle station. He had an anxious look on his face and was a bit short of breath. But he looked up at me and, with an infectious laugh, he said, "Oh, I'm fine. My legs are just old!"

Little information is available about the elderly cardiac rehabilitation patient population. As you read this book, I believe it will become apparent that some of what we do with younger patients in regard to exercise testing and exercise training can be appropriate for elderly patients, but the techniques employed truly become an art form. Thus, many references will be provided on general methods of exercise testing and training that can be used in this patient population. The focus of this book is the art as well as the science of modifying programs to more ideally suit the elderly.

Although exercise testing has been employed in elderly cardiac patients for some time, relatively little information specifically describes the effects of exercise training in this population. There are many more questions than answers about exercise training and lifestyle modification for elderly cardiac patients. Furthermore, our methods for both testing and training this ever-changing population must continually be revised. We are challenged as health professionals to identify appropriate evaluation procedures and training regimens specifically designed for the elderly cardiac patient. This book provides cardiac rehabilitation professionals with a summary of the scientific basis for exercise testing and training of elderly cardiac patients and serves as a practical guide to the operations of these areas.

I hope that this book will be a reference source for those rehabilitation professionals who are beginning to work with the elderly cardiac population. I also hope it will stimulate those rehabilitation professionals currently working with the elderly to evaluate and study their own programs and share their experiences.

Acknowledgments

I would like to gratefully acknowledge the contributions of mentors and colleagues to this work, including Dr. Gene Adams, who got me to begin thinking more seriously about exercise and the elderly; Dr. Phil Wilson, who introduced me to cardiac rehabilitation; Dr. Paul Fardy, without whose personal support, this monograph would not have been possible; and to Dr. Michael Sketch, chief of cardiology at the Creighton University School of Medicine, for all his professional support. Additional thanks to Drs. Dennis Esterbrooks, Kris Berg, Vito Angelillo, Chandra Nair, Dan Hilleman, and Bill Jeffries for their reviews of various sections, to the staff of the Cardiovascular Disease Prevention and Rehabilitation Program at Creighton for their many hours of dedication to patient care, and to Cheri Annin and Stephanie Rockwell for their assistance with the preparation of the manuscript.

Chapter 1

Introduction

The elderly are the fastest growing age group in the United States. Although there is no specific age range for defining *elderly*, between 65 and 74 years of age is commonly used. Those 75 years of age or greater are referred to as *older elderly*. Individuals join the ranks of the elderly at the rate of approximately 1,000 per day, and that number is likely to increase because the average life expectancy for persons reaching age 65 is now more than 80 years (68, 143). In 1991 there were 30 million persons over age 65 in the United States, and this figure is expected to increase to almost 50 million by the year 2020 (20% of the population) (90, 184). Those aged 85 or greater number 3 million at present and are expected to reach 16 million by the year 2030.

The current 12% of the population considered elderly use 30% of all health care resources and a much larger proportion of cardiovascular disease resources. Nearly one half of persons aged 65 or older have cardiovascular disease; coronary artery disease (CAD) is the most common cause of death in the elderly. The prevalence of CAD is greatest (and is similar) in women and men by age 70 (26, 194, 265). The mean age of coronary care unit myocardial infarction patients is now greater than 65 (184). One third of cardiac operations in adults are performed in patients aged 65 or greater (214).

The term *aging* is often used to describe the biological, psychological, and sociological changes that occur in persons over time. It is associated with a decline of the body's functional capacities and a reduction in the system's resistance to disease. Physicians and health care providers for older patients frequently find functional impairment, physical disability, and maintenance of patient independence to be the most challenging problems associated with this age group. However, given the proper health care and the special care that their complex needs require, elderly persons can be healthy and can experience fulfilling lives.

Although the physical and mental manifestations of aging are inevitable, the signs of aging can be offset. An intervention, such as physical activity, that can improve and maintain functional capacity and thereby diminish dependence and disability in older cardiac patients should have important public health implications.

Adults have been encouraged to become physically active by the American Heart Association, the American College of Sports Medicine, the President's Council on Physical Fitness and Sports, and the American Association of Retired Persons. But more than for other age groups, activity programs for the elderly cardiac patient must be tailored to the individual's age, fitness level, and health status, and these vary widely among the elderly (90). The elderly should not be treated as a homogeneous group. In addition, many elderly cardiac patients have one or more chronic diseases that can affect functional capacity. It is not uncommon for elderly cardiac patients to have significant peripheral vascular disease, pulmonary disease, arthritis, and other problems. The altered cardiac structure and functional changes associated with aging, as well as inactivity and deconditioning, also contribute to cardiovascular disability. Limiting the deterioration of functional capacity is a prerequisite to enabling preservation of an independent, active, and energetic lifestyle. Attaining this objective is the goal of the physical activity component of cardiac rehabilitation programs for elderly patients.

Practitioners of exercise prescription for elderly patients must be aware that exercise testing and prescription for the elderly cardiac patient is more of an art than a science. There is much to be learned about appropriate testing methodologies and about adaptation to exercise training in this age group and how best to achieve the maximum benefits of exercise while maintaining safety. The vast differences among individuals will dictate individual exercise prescription methods. Although there are some similarities, one should not expect to routinely observe similar exercise responses in younger and older patients. But it is apparent that improvements in endurance and functional capacity can be achieved with exercise training in cardiac elderly patients. So an understanding of acute and chronic exercise for the elderly cardiac patient is important and requires knowledge of the effects of and interactions between the normal aging process and cardiovascular disease.

Chapter 2

Anatomical and Physiological Considerations: Effects of Aging and Cardiovascular Disease

Although the prevalence of cardiovascular disease increases dramatically with increasing age, aging and disease are not synonymous (100). Whereas aging in itself may cause no disability, its effect can alter the anatomical and physiological settings in which cardiovascular diseases may then develop. And the clinical presentations of the disease processes often change significantly with advancing age.

The marked prevalence of coronary artery disease in the elderly is demonstrated by postmortem studies that show that 60% of people dying from all causes have significant coronary narrowing in at least one major coronary vessel (93). This percentage seems to level off at 50 to 59 years in men and almost two decades later in women (2, 100, 269). Epidemiological studies of persons aged 32 to 90 have found, based on medical histories and resting electrocardiograms, that the prevalence of coronary artery disease ranges from 2% to 30% (153), but these results must be interpreted as indicating only the prevalence of symptomatic coronary artery disease (100). The true prevalence of coronary artery disease includes individuals with *silent* disease as well as those who are symptomatic.

Although the relationship between aging and the incidence of silent myocardial ischemia in the elderly has not yet been thoroughly defined, as much as 75% of the total ischemic time in patients with stable coronary artery disease is asymptomatic, and this percentage may be greater in the elderly (75, 115, 173,

3

217). The following are possible explanations for this increase: The elderly may have an altered perception to pain stimuli, they may have a poor understanding of symptoms, and their presentation of symptoms is more frequently atypical (31, 125–127, 247). Atypical characteristics associated with myocardial ischemia and infarction in the elderly include dyspnea, pulmonary edema, syncope, peripheral arterial embolism, stroke, progressive renal failure, profound weakness, faintness, worsening heart failure, agitation or restlessness, acute confusion or altered mental status, change in eating habits, and other sudden changes in activity or behavior patterns (266).

Structural Changes in the Heart

The major limitation in attempting to describe structural changes in the heart associated with aging is that most studies have included persons with cardiovascular disease; so changes associated with aging may be related, at least in part, to cardiovascular pathology. Nevertheless, in studies of healthy men and women, an aging-related increase in left ventricular wall thickness has been found between the second and seventh decades of life (100, 112, 236). Ventricular hypertrophy usually occurs in response to an increased cardiac volume or afterload. Because no evidence has suggested an increase in resting stroke volume or cardiac output with aging, one must consider increased afterload resulting from increased peripheral resistance as the mechanism for ventricular hypertrophy. It has been recognized that both systolic and mean blood pressures increase with aging at rest and during exercise. However, the degree of left ventricular hypertrophy seen with advancing age is mild compared to that seen in pathological conditions (100, 236).

In addition to structural alterations, common pathological changes have been described in the elderly heart (100). Deposits of adipose between muscle cells are common. The cardiac valves generally thicken. Calcium deposition is frequently noted in the aortic valve and mitral anulus and may result in clinically significant pathology (181, 183).

Systolic and Diastolic Function

Several studies have indicated that resting cardiac output and stroke volume decline with aging. These investigations are difficult to interpret because of the studies' different population characteristics, including a failure to screen for presence or absence of coronary artery disease (100). Nonetheless, cardiac output decreases an average of 1% per year from a mean of 6.5 L·min^{-1} in the third decade to a mean of 3.9 L·$^{-1}$ in the ninth decade (48, 100). Resting stroke volume has been observed to fall 30%, from 85 to 60 ml (48, 157).

In contrast, data from subjects carefully screened for the presence of coronary artery disease demonstrated that resting cardiac function does not decline between the ages of 25 and 80 (209). Further, it has been demonstrated that resting stroke volume does not decline with age (100). Because resting heart rate is also not age-related, these data suggest that resting cardiac output does not decline with increasing age in healthy individuals. Other work using the measurement of the velocity of circumferential fiber shortening in the assessment of intrinsic cardiac muscle function also indicates that this variable is not age-related at rest, again implying that resting cardiac muscle performance is not affected by aging (100, 112).

During exercise, elderly persons performing light work loads achieve stroke volumes similar to those of younger subjects, but smaller increases in stroke volume are observed with increasing work loads. Increases in heart rate and stroke volume are possible during minimal increases in activity with proportional increases in cardiac output. However, the maximum cardiac output in a 65-year-old person is 20% to 30% less than that in a young adult (223). Decreases in both maximal heart rate and maximal stroke volume contribute to the decrease in maximal cardiac output. The ejection fraction increases in younger subjects with increasing exercise; in contrast, older subjects have less increase, with many developing regional ventricular wall motion abnormalities. Higher left ventricular end-diastolic pressure in elderly subjects during exercise has also been documented.

In contrast to systolic function, early left ventricular diastolic function is significantly reduced with increasing age (109, 112). This impairment may be related in part to the previously mentioned age-related increase in left ventricular wall thickness, which would diminish ventricular diastolic compliance (100). Doppler echocardiography has confirmed an age-related slowing of maximal early diastolic mitral inflow (176). Although the reduced filling rate of the elderly heart may not impair resting cardiac performance, it may compromise stroke volume, and therefore cardiac output, when diastolic filling time is shortened during exercise (100).

Peripheral Vasculature

Age-related changes in the blood vessels may limit cardiac performance (100). Pulse wave velocity has been found to increase with age in humans, indicating decreased arterial compliance (22, 100).Structural changes in the aorta and other large arteries are partially reflected clinically by a rise in systolic blood pressure and a widening of pulse pressure with advancing age (100). Evidence suggests that resistance to ventricular emptying increases with aging. Hemodynamic changes occurring in the elderly heart due to increased aortic stiffness require greater left ventricular work and result in increased wall tension and myocardial oxygen consumption during systole. This may explain, in part, the age-related increase in left ventricular mass previously described (100).

Conduction System and Electrocardiogram

With advancing age, there are significant anatomical changes in all parts of the conduction system that can affect physiology. Fat accumulates around the sinoatrial (SA) node, sometimes producing a partial or complete separation of the node from the atrial musculature, which may be related to the development of sick sinus syndrome (100). After age 60, there is a decrease in the number of pacemaker cells in the SA node and by age 75, less than 10% of the cell number found in the young adult remains. In addition, the atrioventricular (A-V) node, the A-V bundle bifurcation, and the proximal left and right bundle branches may become damaged, resulting in idiopathic block (100).

When one considers the anatomical and physiological changes associated with aging, it is not surprising that several features of the electrocardiogram are also altered with aging. Although resting heart rate is not aging-related, PR and QT intervals increase with aging (71, 100, 235). In addition, a leftward shift of the QRS axis occurs. QRS voltage declines with age despite echocardiographic evidence of increased left ventricular mass (100). This has been explained by extracardiac factors such as changes in the heart's position in the thorax, senile emphysema, chest wall deformities, and partial replacement of cardiac muscle by fat (100). However, ST-segment sagging and diminished T-wave amplitude are the most obvious age-related electrocardiographic changes (235).

The prevalence of cardiac arrhythmias at rest and during activity has been found to increase with aging (100, 146). In one study of healthy elderly persons, isolated supraventricular and ventricular ectopic beats were observed in 88% and 78%, respectively (101). Supraventricular tachyarrhythmias were present in one third of the subjects. Twenty-six percent displayed more than 100 supraventricular ectopic beats, and 17% displayed more than 100 ventricular ectopic beats during a 24-hr monitoring period. Ventricular couplets or short runs of ventricular tachycardia were detected in 15%. In each instance, the prevalence was higher than in healthy young subjects reported by other investigators (100). In contrast, atrial fibrillation, sinus bradycardia, sinus pauses, and high-degree A-V block were uncommon. However, results from other investigations have suggested atrial fibrillation is a relatively common arrhythmia in the elderly. Ambulatory studies have indicated that up to 5% of individuals aged 65 or older experience paroxysmal chronic atrial fibrillation. Up to 15% of hospitalized elderly persons experience this arrhythmia (56, 141).

Maximal Oxygen Uptake

Over the last four decades, many studies have shown an aging-related decline in maximal oxygen uptake averaging about 9% per decade between ages 25 and 75 (80, 100, 226). This decline parallels reduced maximal work capacity. It may be largely secondary to a diminished total body muscle mass. The aging-related decline in maximal oxygen uptake has been attributed to a decrease in both maximal cardiac output and maximal arterial venous oxygen ([a-v]O_2) difference (63, 100, 116, 144). Microstructural changes including myofilament disorganization and changes in mitochondrial structure and distribution, which result in reduced oxidative capacity, may explain the reduced maximal (a-v)O_2 difference (226). The physical limitations resulting from a sedentary lifestyle and disabling diseases such as arthritis may also play a role in limiting maximal exercise oxygen uptake (99, 135).

Regarding varying levels of maximal oxygen uptake observed in the elderly, gerontologists have commonly distinguished three categories of senior citizens:

1. *Older elderly* persons, those 75 years of age or greater
2. *Elderly* persons, those 65 to 74 years of age
3. *Athletic-elderly* persons, those who have maintained a high level of fitness throughout life regardless of age

Older elderly persons can reach a maximal oxygen uptake of 2 to 4 METs (1 MET is the resting oxygen uptake while sitting, approximately 3.5 ml of oxygen uptake per kilogram of body weight per minute [ml·kg^{-1}·min^{-1}]). Elderly persons can be expected to attain maximal oxygen uptakes of 5 to 7 METs (17.5 to 24.5 [ml·kg^{-1}·min^{-1}]), and the athletic-elderly have been observed to achieve maximal oxygen uptakes of greater than 10 METs (35 [ml·kg^{-1}·min^{-1}]) (90).

Heart Rate and Blood Pressure

As suggested previously, the resting heart rate generally shows little alteration with aging, although a decline of approximately 1 beat per year during adulthood is seen in the maximal heart rate with exertion (223). The equation

$$220 - age \ (in \ years) = maximal \ heart \ rate$$

has been used to estimate maximal heart rate, although recent literature has shown that many healthy older persons can achieve heart rates higher than those predicted (228). The drop in maximal heart rate with aging results in a 30% to 50% reduction in maximal exercise cardiac output between ages 25 and 85 years (48). Also, the postexertion rate of return to baseline of heart rate, blood pressure, and oxygen consumption are slower for elderly subjects (226).

Changes in blood pressure from rest to exercise are also different for the elderly. Systolic blood pressure is generally higher at rest and during submaximal exercise by as much as 40 mmHg compared to younger adults (84, 157).

Pulmonary System

With aging, lung compliance increases while the ability to expand the chest cavity is impaired (175). Residual volume increases by 30% to 50% as vital capacity decreases by 40% to 50% by age 70 (90, 239). With exertion, the elderly person primarily increases respiratory frequency to increase ventilation rather than increasing depth of respiration. The net effect is an increase of about 20% in work of the respiratory muscles (84).

Nervous System

The important aging-related changes in the central and peripheral nervous systems include slower conduction velocities and reaction times by up to 15% (90). These changes affect the ability to exercise. Both the incidence of sensory deficits and the threshold of perception for many stimuli increase. Changes such as these may be related to the 35% to 40% increase in falls by persons over age 60 (223, 226).

Metabolism

Several metabolic changes occur with aging (90): The basal metabolic rate gradually decreases (226), glucose tolerance diminishes (210), and relative body fat increases as lean body mass decreases (189). Total cholesterol and low density lipoprotein levels increase with aging, whereas the concentration of high density lipoprotein remains unchanged (223).

Muscle and Bone

Changes in the musculoskeletal system occur with alarming frequency in the elderly. Aging is associated with decrements in muscle mass, both in muscle fiber size and number (90, 99). Functionally, muscle strength decreases 20% from age 20 to age 65 (147). In sedentary older adults, the loss of muscle mass and strength may be as great as 40%. As a result, the elderly must use a high proportion of available muscle mass for exercise, which may result in overuse and strain. Clinically, decreased strength and speed of contraction and early onset of fatigue are observed.

Aging is also associated with changes in the connective tissues (137). Connective tissues, including fascia, ligaments, and tendons, become less extensible. Range of motion, both active and passive, declines with advancing years, but it is not clear whether this decreased flexibility results from biological aging, degenerative disease, inactivity, or some combination of these factors (90). Degeneration of the joints, especially the spine, is often found in elderly persons (135). Weight-bearing activity may accelerate this onset; non-weight-bearing exercise training to promote strength gains may decelerate it (99, 135).

There is progressive bone loss with aging (90). Women over age 35 lose bone mass at a rate of about 1% per year. Men begin bone loss at about age 55 and lose 10% to 15% by age 70 (8, 238). Decreasing dietary calcium intake, diabetes mellitus, renal impairment, and immobilization may accelerate bone loss. The resulting loss of bone strength predisposes the elderly to fractures, which are a significant cause of morbidity and mortality in the elderly.

Summary

In deriving conclusions about the effects of aging on cardiovascular performance during exercise, and subsequently, the potential long-term benefits of exercise training, one should keep in mind that cardiovascular disease, specifically heart disease, was probably present in a significant number of the older individuals evaluated in early studies, as suggested by the sizable proportion of these subjects with electrocardiographic abnormalities. Also, acute responses to submaximal and maximal exercise may have been affected in these investigations by noncardiovascular factors such as physical activity status and respiratory function (just to mention two possibilities). Thus, conclusions about the limits in cardiovascular performance imposed by aging must be tentative. Additional study is warranted of both healthy elderly subjects and those with cardiovascular disease (100).

Chapter 3

Exercise Testing

Exercise testing is a valuable tool for assessing the cardiovascular system (136). Exercise testing uses the physiological changes that occur during physical activity to create an altered hemodynamic state to which the cardiovascular, pulmonary, and muscular systems must respond (26). Most exercise testing protocols involve dynamic exercise during which the heart rate and systolic blood pressure normally increase while diastolic blood pressure remains constant or demonstrates a modest decrease. An increase in the work of the heart is represented by an elevation of the heart rate × systolic blood pressure, or rate pressure product (RPP), corresponding to an increase in myocardial oxygen demand. Autonomic regulation and the accumulation of myocardial metabolic by-products are associated with coronary vasodilatation and a concomitant increase in coronary artery blood flow. When coronary stenoses are present, obstruction to flow may lead to a demand-supply imbalance of oxygenated blood to the myocardium, resulting in exercise-induced myocardial ischemia. In elderly cardiac patients, as in younger patients, exercise testing can also be useful in determining functional capacity, detecting arrhythmias, evaluating therapeutic interventions, and determining prognosis (10, 26, 79).

Methodology

The basic applications of exercise testing have been described elsewhere (58, 91, 106, 249). Indications for exercise testing of the elderly cardiac patient are similar to those for younger patients and include risk stratification, assessment of functional capacity, efficacy of medical or surgical interventions, exercise prescription, and increasing patient's and family's confidence about health status and activity levels. The primary differences concern the modifications and special

11

considerations needed to accomplish the testing objectives in this patient group. This section emphasizes these considerations.

Selection of Appropriate Patients for Testing

The screening of elderly cardiac patients for appropriateness of testing, particularly noting the presence or absence of postinfarction angina or signs or symptoms of left ventricular failure, is an essential part of obtaining reliable information and ensuring safety. Contraindications for exercise testing in the elderly include unstable angina pectoris, acute congestive heart failure, uncontrolled arrhythmias, advanced heart block, severe aortic stenosis and mitral stenosis, acute myocarditis or pericarditis, recent pulmonary emboli, resting hypertension (greater than 180/100 mmHg), and inability to exercise. Determining whether the elderly cardiac patient is capable of performing the exercise test is also a criterion for risk stratification (78, 105). Elderly postmyocardial infarction patients who are ineligible for predischarge exercise testing on the basis of clinical profile and resting ejection fraction have a 1-year mortality rate approaching 40%, compared to 4% in those eligible for testing. However, as important as these contraindications are, other cardiovascular, neurological, and musculoskeletal conditions in the elderly cardiac patient may preclude testing or the adequate performance of an exercise test.

Performance may also be limited by fear and anxiety. Problems peculiar to the elderly cardiac patient may occur during exercise testing, and it is critical that cardiac rehabilitation professionals be aware of them (255). These potential problems—including early appearance of fatigue and light-headedness due to muscular weakness and deconditioning or vasoregulatory insufficiency—will affect the outcome of the exercise test and should be considered prior to initiating the referral for exercise testing. When the decision is made to perform this evaluation, these patients may require a more detailed explanation and a demonstration of procedures prior to testing as well as physical or emotional support during testing (161). Testing should be tailored to meet the needs of the elderly cardiac patient while obtaining an optimal amount of clinical information.

Safety Precautions

To obtain the diagnostic and prognostic advantages of exercise testing and to ensure safety, those supervising exercise tests in elderly cardiac patients should be aware of the patients' possible exercise responses and reasons for test discontinuation (205). Those reasons include progressive angina, complex ventricular arrhythmias, exertional hypotension (greater than or equal to 20 mmHg), horizontal or downsloping ST-segment depression equal to or greater than 3 mm, onset of advanced heart block, onset of severe exercise hypertension, failure of appropriate chronotropic increase, neuromuscular discoordination or other signs of inappropriate circulatory adjustments, musculoskeletal discomfort, and request by subject to stop.

The American Heart Association has provided explicit safety precautions for exercise testing laboratories (249). Everything necessary for cardiopulmonary resuscitation must be available, and regular drills should be performed to make certain that both personnel and equipment are ready for a cardiac emergency. A survey of clinical exercise facilities has shown that exercise testing is safe, with not more than 1 death and 5 nonfatal complications per 10,000 tests (106). The literature contains reports of acute myocardial infarctions and death occurring secondary to this procedure, but with appropriate screening these can probably be avoided. Unfortunately, little information is available on the safety of exercise testing for the elderly cardiac population. Rehabilitation professionals can reduce the number of emergent events associated with exercise testing in this population by determining the appropriateness of testing through a thorough screening, being knowledgeable about expected responses to exercise in this population and indications for the cessation of the exercise test, and implementing all precautions necessary for personnel and equipment.

Treadmill Testing

This modality is the most common form of exercise testing in the United States primarily because of its ease of administration and the familiarity of subjects with the type of exercise employed (i.e., walking). Also, it may have a greater appeal in terms of program marketing and public perception of credibility than a bicycle ergometer (26). Elderly cardiac patients, however, may feel uncertain and unsteady on a treadmill because of problems related to balance, joint stiffness, or other musculoskeletal limitations that reduce their ability to perform standard treadmill protocols. Elderly patients may hang on to the handrails and use them for an undue amount of support, thus making the predicted oxygen requirements for the various treadmill protocols less valid. It is particularly important when testing the elderly patient on a treadmill to provide a period of familiarization with this device prior to the actual exercise test, using work loads of 1 to 1.2 miles per hour with no grade. Also, an elderly cardiac patient's physical capacity may be less than the stress imposed by the first stage or two of some standard testing protocols. If this is suspected, a protocol should be used that begins at a lower work load and increases more gradually, such as those used for testing after myocardial infarction. The initial work load should not exceed 3 METs unless the testing staff is familiar with the patient's capabilities. Higher work loads may be supramaximal. In addition, treadmill protocols that require elderly cardiac patients to exercise at speeds greater than 4 miles per hour may be particularly difficult. Suggested treadmill exercise protocols for the elderly patient include the modified Bruce, Naughton, and Balke protocols (see Table 3.1).

Bicycle Ergometer

The bicycle ergometer may provide an effective alternative for elderly cardiac patients with fear of falling or unsteadiness in walking, for those who are obese, and for those with musculoskeletal problems that preclude sustained unsupported

Table 3.1   Exercise Testing Protocols for Elderly Cardiac Patients

Protocol	Stage	Work load	Estimated MET level
Balke (249)	1	3 mph, 0% grade	3
	2	3 mph, 2% grade	4
	3	3 mph, 5% grade	5
	4	3 mph, 7.5% grade	6
	5	3 mph, 10% grade	7
	6	3 mph, 12.5% grade	8
Modified Bruce (221)	1	1.7 mph, 0% grade	2.3
	2	1.7 mph, 5% grade	3.5
	3	1.7 mph, 10% grade	4.8
	4	2.5 mph, 12% grade	6.6
	5	3.4 mph, 14% grade	8.4
	6	4.2 mph, 16% grade	10.2
Naughton (186)	1	2 mph, 0% grade	2
	2	2 mph, 3.5% grade	3
	3	2 mph, 7% grade	4
	4	2 mph, 10.5% grade	5
	5	2 mph, 14% grade	6
	6	2 mph, 17.5% grade	7
Bicycle ergometer (249)	1	150 kgm	2.4
	2	300 kgm	3.7
	3	450 kgm	4.9
	4	600 kgm	6.1
	5	750 kgm	7.3
	6	900 kgm	8.5
Air-Dyne (arms alone) (24)	1	.5 Air-Dyne units	2.6
	2	1.0 Air-Dyne units	4.4
	3	1.5 Air-Dyne units	5.8
	4	2.0 Air-Dyne units	7.2
	5	2.5 Air-Dyne units	8.7
	6	3.0 Air-Dyne units	10.1

walking (26). Bicycle testing protocols have several advantages and disadvantages. Elderly cardiac patients often feel more secure sitting in a stable position, and the bicycle ergometer provides the patient with added control for discontinuing the test. But because the muscles used in bicycle exercise are often not well conditioned, early test discontinuation may ensue from local muscle fatigue. Also, limitations in neuromuscular coordination and limited recent bicycling experience may lead to erratic pedaling speed, which is a problem for those using mechanically braked ergometers. These can be major limiting factors for bicycle testing. Electronically braked ergometers may reduce the impact of these problems, but they are often difficult to calibrate, potentially providing a different source of work load variability. As with treadmill testing, and because of frequently deconditioned muscles in the lower extremities, initial work loads and increments of work load increases should be reduced in tests of the elderly cardiac patient. Additionally, exercise stages of 2 to 3 min in duration beginning at a work load not exceeding 25 W and increasing by increments not exceeding 25 W should be considered. One additional note is that cycling can generate greater blood pressure increases than walking, owing to the development of muscle tension in the thighs.

Arm Ergometry

Elderly cardiac patients who have vascular, neurological, or orthopedic impairment of lower extremities may be candidates for upper extremity exercise testing (26). Most upper extremity protocols use an arm ergometer, and most involve arm cranking at incremental work loads of 10 to 25 W for 2- or 3-min stages. Arm ergometry testing requires that special care be taken to place electrodes just below the clavicles to ensure stable lead positions. Blood pressure measurement is also difficult and may dictate that the patient either stop exercising or drop one arm while continuing to crank with the other arm. Dropping the arm may require the test technician to assist with cranking momentarily. A discontinuous exercise protocol for arm testing may allow greater exercise capacity and cardiovascular end points (heart rate, blood pressure, and myocardial oxygen demand) to be obtained while providing a mechanism for improved electrocardiograms and blood pressure measurements. Rest periods of 30 s to 2 min are suggested between work loads. A successful protocol very much depends on subject motivation, and this is particularly true in elderly cardiac patients. Unfortunately, elderly cardiac patients who are too weak or debilitated to perform treadmill or bicycle exercise are often unable to adequately perform an arm ergometry test. Performance of arm tests in these cases often results in reduced cardiovascular responses, thus decreasing the sensitivity of the exercise test.

Skin Preparation

Proper skin preparation is essential for good results in an exercise test (106). Because electrical noise increases during testing, it is crucial to lower the resistance at the skin-electrode interface and thereby improve the signal-to-noise ratio. It is important that the exercise test technician prepare the skin consistently and thoroughly even though the patient may experience some mild discomfort or minor skin irritation. Performing an exercise test with an electrocardiographic signal that cannot be continuously monitored and accurately interpreted because of artifact is useless and dangerous.

The areas for electrode application should be marked with a felt-tip pen, the marks serving as a guide for removal of enough of the superficial layer of the skin to reduce the signal-to-noise ratio (106). Usually the electrodes are placed using anatomical landmarks that are found with the patient in the supine position, but some elderly individuals with loose skin can have significant shift of electrode positions when they assume an upright position. In these cases, anatomical landmarks used for electrode placement should be made while the patient is upright. The marked areas are then cleansed with an alcohol-saturated gauze pad. The next step is to remove the superficial layer of skin either with a hand-held, battery-driven instrument or by abrasion with fine-grain emery paper. The skin of an elderly patient is delicate and should be prepped carefully. Ultimately, a careful preparation saves time by reducing the frequency of test interruptions due to significant artifact in the tracings.

Maximal Oxygen Uptake

Maximal oxygen uptake has been suggested to be the best single indicator of fitness. Direct assessment of expired gases may provide insight into the physiological limitations observed at maximal exercise and may be particularly beneficial in assessing the effects of exercise training in the elderly population. However, few data are available describing the direct measurement of oxygen uptake in elderly cardiac patients, primarily because it is often thought to be clinically impractical, particularly in the elderly cardiac patient (4). Many elderly cardiac patients find the task of exercising maximally challenging enough without the introduction of a rather cumbersome mouthpiece and nose clip. Also, testers may find it difficult to obtain appropriate verbal information from elderly patients while obtaining direct measurements. If direct assessment of maximal oxygen uptake is undertaken, it may be helpful to provide tables and charts to which a patient can refer to describe symptoms or perception of effort (see Tables 3.2 and 3.3). For the angina scale, the patient would be asked to point at the number that corresponds to the severity of chest discomfort. For the rating of perceived exertion scale, the patient would indicate a number describing his or her perception of total body exertion, not focusing on any one area of the body. Other disadvantages of the maximal oxygen uptake test include the additional expense of equipment and supplies and the necessity for appropriately trained technical staff with a good understanding of exercise physiology.

Table 3.2   Angina Scale

Rating	Description of pain intensity
1+	Light, barely noticeable
2+	Moderate, bothersome
3+	Severe, very uncomfortable
4+	Most severe pain ever experienced

From *Guidelines for Exercise Testing and Prescription* (4th ed.) (p. 73) by the American College of Sports Medicine, 1991, Philadelphia: Lea & Febiger. Copyright 1991 by Lea & Febiger. Reprinted by permission.

Table 3.3   Rating of Perceived Exertion (RPE)

Numerical rating	Description of perceived level of effort
6	
7	Very, very light
8	
9	Very light
10	
11	Fairly light
12	
13	Somewhat hard
14	
15	Hard
16	
17	Very hard
18	
19	Very, very hard
20	

From "Perceived Exertion as an Indicator of Somatic Stress" by G. Borg, 1970, *Scandinavian Journal of Rehabilitation Medicine*, 2, p. 93. Copyright 1970 by Gunnar Borg. Reprinted by permission.

For some or all of these reasons, most data on oxygen uptake values resulting from clinical exercise testing in elderly cardiac patients are derived using estimation equations based on specific testing protocols. The ease with which testing can be performed using oxygen uptake estimation equations is attractive and, in most casts, preferred. But such equations have limitations. Most of the equations and resulting normative values for maximal oxygen uptake have been derived based on measured responses in younger subjects, so these estimations may not accurately reflect values for elderly cardiac patients. Using these equations often results in overestimations of oxygen uptake in these patients. The contrasts between values obtained through direct assessment and those derived through the use of equations probably result from a combination of the effects of ischemic heart disease, the cardiovascular and oxygen kinetics responses to exercise in the elderly compared to younger patients, and the potential neuromuscular discoordination that may lead to either patients' having to work excessively hard to accomplish the task of walking or patients' having to hold on to the handrails. One must consider the advantages as well as the limitations of each maximal oxygen uptake assessment technique when deciding on a standard method.

Postexercise Period of Recovery

The patient should be supine in the postexercise period for maximal test sensitivity (106). But it is advisable to record an electrocardiogram while the patient stands motionless (sits motionless if using bicycle or arm ergometry) immediately after the test while the patient still has a near-maximal heart rate. The patient should then be moved quickly to the supine position. This can increase end-diastolic volume because venous return is enhanced as the patient assumes the supine position. The increased end-diastolic volume may increase the work of the heart due to increased wall stress, thus increasing myocardial oxygen demand. This may cause or exacerbate signs or symptoms associated with ischemia, including depth of the ST-segment depression or severity of angina pectoris. Some exercise testing laboratories may require that patients experiencing ischemic signs or symptoms be asked to sit for 1 to 2 min to avoid exacerbation of these results.

Some patients must lie down immediately to avoid symptoms associated with postexercise hypotension or neuromuscular discoordination resulting from the treadmill coming to a halt or the sudden cessation of movement. Such neuromuscular discoordination is often observed in the elderly; test supervisory personnel should carefully observe these patients in order to reduce the potential for falls at times of speed and grade changes, and particularly as the patient moves to the supine position at the end of exercise. The elderly cardiac patient may be more likely to experience an increase in dyspnea following the cessation of exercise testing as he or she moves into the supine position. Consequently, it may be appropriate to have some patients simply sit for the first minute or two of recovery before moving them into the supine position. Patient monitoring should continue each minute for at least 6 min postexercise or until exercise responses have returned to baseline. Observation of the patient should not be limited to watching patient monitors and looking for adverse signs and symptoms during and at the end of exercise.

Interpretation of Results

Although exercise testing is the principle noninvasive method for determining cardiovascular status and disease in younger age groups, there is disagreement about its efficacy in elderly cardiac patients (255). But as with any mode of medical testing, patients must be evaluated as individuals, not as members of an arbitrary age group. There is no evidence that age alone increases the risk of exercise testing; however, the significance of some findings in the elderly population varies from that of younger individuals. For example, ST-segment depression or exercise dyspnea may have different predictive values in the elderly. This section describes findings resulting from exercise testing in the elderly cardiac population.

Exercise Capacity

Reduced functional capacity—brought on largely by a sedentary lifestyle and physical problems peculiar to the elderly, as well as by cardiovascular disease—frequently limits exercise test performance (255). In fact, data collected from elderly cardiac patients suggest that this group's exercise capacity when undergoing maximal testing if often limited by noncardiopulmonary factors (4). Limiting factors such as dyspnea, fear of overexertion, muscular weakness, inflexibility, and poor motivation may be more prevalent in older than in younger cardiac patients. Many exercise protocols do not adequately consider these factors; therefore, older patients frequently become fatigued before maximum cardiovascular end points are achieved. Data suggest that peak oxygen uptake in elderly cardiac patients is not synonymous with *maximal* oxygen uptake. This does not necessarily imply an increased risk of future cardiac events (59, 255). Therefore, reduced exercise duration may not be as ominous in older persons unless other significant abnormalities such as ST-segment depression, angina, or complex arrhythmias are observed.

Exercise Heart Rate

The mechanism of decline in maximal heart rate with increasing age is uncertain (128, 162). Many factors may be involved: sympathetic and parasympathetic drive mechanisms, increased duration of isovolumic relaxation time, the patient's fear of severe exercise or lack of motivation, caution on the part of the test supervisory staff, or simply the inability to exercise to a great enough intensity because of deconditioning, musculoskeletal limitations, or increased prevalence and severity of peripheral vascular disease. Also, there may be a direct effect of the aging process on the sinoatrial node, resulting in chronotropic incompetence.

One goal of an exercise test is to obtain a near-maximal heart rate response for the subject's age. However, the mean percentage of maximal heart rate recorded in elderly cardiac patients varies from 75% to 97% of the maximum predicted heart rate for age (4, 5, 277, 278, 279). In addition to the reasons mentioned in the previous paragraph, this may in part be secondary to beta-blocker therapy (4, 255, 278). Table 3.4 illustrates the peak exercise heart rate, blood pressure, and rate pressure product responses of elderly cardiac patients obtained during exercise testing at various stages of recovery from myocardial infarction or coronary artery bypass graft surgery. The combination of a failure to achieve an adequate rate pressure product and a reduced maximal exercise capacity has been associated with a poor prognosis in elderly cardiac patients (98, 215).

Exercise Blood Pressure

As with exercise heart rate during testing, systolic blood pressure rises as work load increases (255). A rising systolic blood pressure during increasing levels of exercise indicates well-preserved left ventricular function and an overall better prognosis (218). But a systolic reading above a maximal range of 220 to 240 mmHg is considered a hypertensive response to exercise. On the other hand, a flat or hypotensive response to exertion, especially manifested at low work loads, suggests a poor prognosis and is usually associated with severe left ventricular dysfunction. This dysfunction is usually ischemic in origin, although in elderly

Table 3.4 Acute Responses to Exercise Testing Performed Pre- and Postexercise Training in Elderly Cardiac Patients

Study	N	Age range in years (mean)	Initial test postevent	Training period	Maximal heart rate (bpm)	Maximal systolic	Rate pressure product ($\times 10^{-2}$)	METs
Williams et al. (278)	76	65–82 (70)	4 weeks	10 weeks	126/138	161/171	205/234	5.3/8.1
Ades et al. (5)	15	62–77 (65)	6 weeks	12 weeks	130/133	152/158	199/224	6.2/10.4
Ades et al. (4)	22	62–77 (68)	8 weeks	12 weeks	133/132	—	—	4.8/6.1
Williams et al. (277)	260	65–74 (69)	4 weeks	10 weeks	129/131	166/171	214/224	3.3/7.0
	56	75–84 (78)			126/129	172/177	217/228	2.9/4.3
Williams et al. (279)	18	65–82 (69)	4 weeks	18 months	122/130	158/166	193/216	4.9/8.6

Note. Data for heart rate, blood pressure, rate pressure product, and METs are pre- and posttraining data (i.e., 126/138 bpm for maximal heart rate represents a heart rate of 126 at maximal exercise on test at program entrance and a heart rate of 138 at follow-up).

patients the higher prevalence of cardiomyopathy, stenotic valvular lesions, and exercise-induced arrhythmias may also account for these findings (255).

Contrary to the normal rise in systolic blood pressure, diastolic blood pressure should remain constant or decrease by 10 to 20 mmHg during dynamic exercise due to the dilatation of the peripheral arterioles of exercising muscle. An increase of more than 10 to 20 mmHg in diastolic blood pressure during exercise is abnormal (49). Exercise-induced elevation of diastolic blood pressure identifies a population with ventricular dysfunction, increased severity of CAD, and increased peripheral vascular resistance (225). Both exercise-induced systolic and diastolic hypertension may be more prevalent in the elderly.

Ventricular Arrhythmias

Exercise-induced ventricular arrhythmias occur in 35% to 50% of healthy middle-aged men, and the incidence increases with age (255). Exercise-induced ventricular arrhythmias occur in 38% to 65% of patients with CAD, and complex arrhythmias occur in 30% (152). In general, patients with CAD manifest arrhythmias at a lower heart rate, and arrhythmias are somewhat more reproducible in these patients than in clinically normal subjects. By themselves, exercise-induced ventricular arrhythmias are not necessarily predictive of future cardiac events, even in patients with CAD. However, when the patient also has ischemic ST-segment depression, these arrhythmias may be predictive of significant multivessel disease and impaired left ventricular function. Complex ventricular arrhythmias in conjunction with an inadequate rise in rate pressure product have been associated with increased risk of future coronary events in the elderly cardiac patient (215). And, in patients who had a recent myocardial infarction or coronary artery bypass graft surgery prior to entrance into early exercise training, the occurrence of complex ventricular arrhythmias during exercise testing has been associated with an increased risk of abnormal electrocardiographic events during early exercise training that require medication change or more significant intervention (274).

ST-Segment Depression

Electrocardiographic evidence of ischemia is classically represented by flat or downsloping ST-segment depression. In the elderly, the significance of ST-segment depression is an important finding. Analysis using Bayes theorem suggests that exercise-induced ST-segment depression may be more significant in the older population than in the young because of the higher prevalence of CAD in older people (85, 148, 256). However, a fairly high incidence of exercise-induced ST-segment depression has been noted in elderly patients without CAD (255). These false-positive responses suggest that ST-segment depression in the elderly is not as specific for CAD but may reflect an increased prevalence of diseases that affect ventricular compliance, which in turn may affect repolarization. The use of cardiac medications in the elderly can also distort test results. For these reasons, exercise-induced ST-segment depression in the elderly is best interpreted in the context of other variables such as angina, arrhythmias, blood pressure response, and exercise tolerance (255). Nevertheless, one should be aware that ST-segment depression following myocardial infarction in elderly patients has been associated with increased risk of future events (114). Also, ST-segment depression during exercise testing in post-myocardial infarction patients, prior to entering into early exercise training, has been associated with an increased risk of abnormal electrocardiographic events during exercise training that require medication change or more significant interventions (274).

The evaluation of other variables, including R-wave and T-wave changes, QT-interval analysis, and the analysis of the ST-segment/heart rate slope to confirm the significance of exercise-induced ST-segment depression may be of some value, but little information is available that is specific to the elderly (156, 255). The significance of ST-segment depression with exercise may be associated with an abnormal increase in the height of the R wave or decrease in the depth of the Q wave.

Angina

Anginal chest discomfort during exercise testing is predictive of the presence and severity of CAD and of the risk for subsequent coronary events in younger individuals (59). The presence of angina pectoris also enhances the predictive significance of ST-segment changes. Unfortunately, symptoms of chest discomfort in elderly cardiac patients are not always clearly anginal in nature. A history of chest discomfort is often vague because older patients lead a more sedentary lifestyle, and hence chest discomfort may not have a prominent exertional component. Furthermore, arthritis, musculoskeletal problems, and claudication are frequent and may limit activity before anginal discomfort occurs. Elderly patients with previously asymptomatic coronary atherosclerosis may have myocardial ischemia or angina precipitated by hypertension, anemia, or arrhythmias (264).

Radionuclide Evaluations

The many confounding variables associated with cardiac disease in the elderly patient suggest that conventional exercise testing may not always be the most useful tool in diagnosing CAD or in making assessment of risk stratification (140). Often the electrocardiogram of the elderly patient is characterized by left ventricular hypertrophy, previous myocardial infarction, effects of digitalis, and nonspecific ST-segment changes. These abnormalities reduce the specificity of the electrocardiographic response to ischemia.

Radionuclide scintigraphy during exercise testing has demonstrated greater sensitivity and specificity for CAD than the electrocardiographic response alone. Specifically, the thallium exercise test has been demonstrated to provide prognostic information particularly applicable to the elderly population (139). In patients over age 65 who perform exercise testing for evaluation of CAD, the presence of a reversible thallium defect has been shown to correspond to an 8% cardiovascular event rate in the following 4 years versus a 1% event rate in those without demonstrable thallium defects (140). But radionuclide scintigraphy, whether using thallium or another radiopharmaceutical agent (sestamibi, teboroxine), requires additional time, expense, equipment, space, and personnel. Exercise echocardiography has been demonstrated to be effective in evaluating coronary heart disease, but little experience is available in the elderly.

Pharmacological stress testing, in conjunction with nuclear scintigraphy utilizing any of several radiopharmaceutical agents, appears particularly well suited for use in the debilitated elderly subject who cannot appropriately perform exercise (32, 111, 248). Intravenous dipyridamole testing appears relatively safe and has a reported sensitivity of 86% and a specificity of 75% for detecting CAD in patients over age 70 (158). Because of the number and severity of side effects, as well as some methodological limitations, pharmacological agents other than dipyridamole used in conjunction with radionuclide imaging, echocardiography, or position emission tomography (PET) have also been investigated (108, 118, 138, 233, 257, 258, 284). In elderly females, the use of adenosine as a cardiac stressor in conjunction with thallium 201 in the evaluation of CAD resulted in improved levels of sensitivity and specificity compared to exercise radionuclide imaging, as well as having a low side-effect profile (273). Thus, early evidence suggests that several pharmacological agents can be effectively used and may provide enhanced levels of specificity and sensitivity in the elderly patient population. The major limitation of pharmacological stress testing in cardiac rehabilitation exercise training is that no information on exercise capacity can be obtained, and thus the relationship of functional capacity and CAD cannot be discerned.

Summary

Exercise testing in elderly cardiac patients has been demonstrated to be useful in measuring functional status relative to the patient's limitations and in evaluating therapeutic interventions. Although some additional considerations are needed in interpreting data of elderly patients compared to that of younger cardiac patients, the use of appropriate modalities and the implementation of individualized techniques will result in obtaining the optimum level of information from this procedure.

Chapter 4

Exercise Prescription

The most critical factor in an elderly cardiac patient's ability to function independently in society is mobility, the ability to move without assistance (90). The overall focus for exercise training should be to improve mobility by enhancing health-related fitness components such as cardiorespiratory and muscular endurance, body composition, flexibility, and strength. Older people who maintain cardiorespiratory fitness and flexibility, as well as a body composition with the appropriate ratio of muscle to fat, retain mobility longer than those who become obese and allow their muscular and cardiorespiratory systems to deteriorate. As is explained in chapter 5, the cardiorespiratory system of the older cardiac patient is capable of exercise training, and good aerobic fitness levels are achievable. Regular exercise can lead to a loss of fat, maintenance of an acceptable body composition, increased strength, and increased muscle mass.

Entering the Program

Two initial steps are necessary for the prescription of exercise: physician referral of the patient and appropriate evaluation of the patient prior to entering the exercise program. As the referral process itself appears to be a primary limitation to elderly patients' participation, several considerations should be made for enhancing this process. Appropriate referral and development of the exercise program based on the evaluation results are critical to establishing patient objectives and implementing the exercise program.

Referral

Elderly cardiac patients, particularly females, have a relatively low rate of entry into exercise training programs. Ades et al. have reported a 20% to 25% entry rate for elderly males, whereas only 15% of eligible female patients were referred into early post-hospital discharge cardiac rehabilitation (Phase II); in younger patients the overall rate was 57% (5, 7). Our own program has entry rates of 25% and 13% among elderly male and female patients, respectively, compared with an overall 74% rate among younger participants (278). Differences in referral rates may reflect the attitudes of the referring physicians, the patients' families, and the participants themselves. The strength of the referring physician's recommendation for participation has been suggested to be the most powerful predictor of patient entrance into the program (7). Issues concerning the patient's accessibility to the program and emotional status at entrance are also important considerations (6). These latter issues may be subject to physician and family attitudes on the patient's entrance into the program. Concomitant illnesses common in the elderly patient population may also preclude participation. The differences in referral rates between elderly males and females, however, do not appear to be due to differences in clinical profiles; no major differences are apparent at program entrance.

Initial Evaluation

The initial evaluation provides information for establishing the goals of an exercise training program. Each patient should have a careful and complete evaluation before his or her exercise training regimen is devised. Chronic diseases should be identified and physical activities appropriately modified to provide for more enjoyable and practical exercise and to avoid injury and exacerbation of underlying conditions (99, 239). Realistic program goals should be established based on the patient's interests and needs. Patient information collected at the initial evaluation may include name, sex, and age; reason for referral; past medical history, including cardiovascular and other significant medical history (myocardial infarction, coronary artery bypass graft surgery, percutaneous transluminal coronary angioplasty, angina, valvular diseases, etc.); date and results of cardiac catheterization; cardiac risk factors; medications; and laboratory findings.

The elderly cardiac patient may have a variety of characteristics that require special consideration. These characteristics concern dietary history, evaluation for sensory deficits, and determination of musculoskeletal abnormalities (99). Dietary inadequacies are prevalent and may be compounded by modest increases in caloric expenditure from exercise training (223). The combination of appropriate diet and exercise is important to achieving several benefits of physical activity. For example, although exercise should improve bone mass, an adequate calcium intake is required to allow an increase rather than a redistribution of bone mineral (240).

Peripheral neuropathy, gait disturbance, impaired equilibrium, or orthostatic hypotension should alert the physician and cardiac rehabilitation staff to an increased potential for falls. Degenerative joint disease is also common in this age group. Assessment of joint stability and range of motion should be performed prior to exercise training, and, when appropriate, activity should be adjusted accordingly (99).

The review of a patient's medication regimen should include consideration of possible interactions with activity programs (90). Diuretics may predispose patients to hypocalcemia, hypokalemia, arrhythmias, and volume depletion. Beta-blocking drugs can alter exercise parameters and reduce exercise tolerance in some elderly individuals, whereas tranquilizers can cause orthostatic dizziness and impair thermoregulation. Patients on insulin or related oral medications may require dose adjustment. Medications and exercise in the elderly are discussed in more detail later in this chapter.

Determining the Exercise Prescription

Aerobic exercise involving the large muscle groups is best for achieving the health and fitness goals of both healthy and cardiac elderly populations (224). The combination of intensity, frequency, duration, and mode of aerobic exercise has been found to be effective in providing a training effect (205, 230). Activities such as walking, jogging, rowing, and swimming are recommended. The use of smaller muscle groups, even in aerobic activity, may result in relatively larger increases in blood pressure and cardiac work at similar exercise work loads. Resistance training or upper extremity aerobic training is generally considered less practical for the elderly. But if an exercise prescription focuses on aerobic exercise involving the lower extremities, such as walking and cycling, a relative weakening of the upper extremity muscles can occur (224). With appropriate precautions and supervision, resistance training, particularly of the upper body, can be of significant value in the elderly patient population for maintaining or increasing strength and muscle mass.

The following are general recommendations for early short-term exercise training (Phase II) in elderly cardiac patients:

- **Intensity**—50% to 80% of the peak oxygen uptake attained at the most recent exercise test corresponding to 60% to 85% of the peak heart rate at the same test
- **Frequency**—Participation in a formal training program 3 days per week, and home exercise (walking or cycle ergometry) 3 to 5 days per week
- **Duration**—55 min per session, including 10 min of warm-up and stretching exercises; 20 to 40 min of aerobic exercise, broken up into shorter periods, allowing for 1- to 2-min rest intervals when appropriate; and 10 min of cool-down and flexibility exercises
- **Mode**—Alternating arm and leg exercise using treadmill walking, leg ergometry, and arm ergometry

In addition to these general guidelines, some specific comments on intensity, frequency, duration, and mode are noteworthy, particularly as the prescription is extended into the long-term training program (Phase III).

Sign- or Symptom-Limited Exercise Testing

The exercise prescription should be based on a pretraining sign- or symptom-limited graded exercise test so that exercise response can be evaluated and appropriate recommendations can be made for heart rate and work load intensity based on peak cardiovascular responses. Maximal exercise intensity and cardiovascular responses during exercise testing are described in chapter 3; typically, elderly cardiac patients entering Phase II exercise training have maximal heart rates from 116 to 136 beats per min and maximal oxygen uptakes from 2 to 5 METs (278). Our experience suggests that less than 25% of elderly patients have exercise capacities greater than 5 METs at Phase II entrance.

Exercise Intensity

The physical work capacity of the elderly cardiac patient, both prior to and following exercise training, is often significantly lower than that observed in younger cardiac patients (278). Because many elderly patients have been sedentary for a long time, specific muscle groups are often severely deconditioned, particularly those used during arm or leg cycle ergometry. This observation provides additional rationale for the musculoskeletal evaluation that should take place during the initial evaluation. Many elderly patients have musculoskeletal limitations that are as limiting or more limiting than their cardiac limitations. For these patients, it is important to prescribe low exercise work load intensities, particularly during the first few weeks of training. Our elderly cardiac patients usually begin training at a 2- to 3-MET level, whereas younger cardiac patients begin at a 3- to 5-MET level (275). Based on 70% of peak exercise test heart rates, the initial mean exercise training target heart rates of elderly patients in our program have been 92 ± 8 beats per min for patients not receiving beta-blocking drugs and 81 ± 10 beats per min for those using beta blockers.

It is not uncommon for elderly cardiac patients in the Phase II program to be incapable of exercising within the recommended intensity range (60% to 85% of peak heart rate). In these instances, patients are encouraged to exercise but at considerably reduced intensities (50% to 60% of peak heart rate). When exercise training intensity is low, participants are encouraged to increase the frequency of exercise, perhaps to even three or four times per day.

When exercise testing has not been performed prior to training, which may be the case for as many as 50% of elderly patients, alternative methods can be used to prescribe exercise. These include the use of reduced exercise work loads and ratings of perceived exertion early in the program. These alternative methods allow the patient to continue to exercise in a supervised setting while the exercise prescription is modified based on the results from several sessions (205). Evaluation should begin at very low work loads (2 to 3 METs) to ensure safety until appropriate safe levels are identified.

Patient progress should be reviewed periodically and the review should include consideration for increasing the exercise training target heart rate. This assessment can be easily accomplished with repeat exercise testing, although this may not be possible for all patients during Phase II because of economic issues and the perceived value of such testing for purposes other than prescribing exercise. Hence, the cardiac rehabilitation staff may need to rely on data collected during the first few weeks of exercise training to provide a means of safely increasing intensity during the latter weeks of Phase II. In general, exercise target heart rates can be increased by 5% of the initial exercise test peak heart rate at 4-week intervals when repeat exercise testing has not been performed. Of course, these increases are made only in patients who have been asymptomatic during training, have not exhibited contraindications to increased exercise intensity, and have shown normal training adaptation.

During long-term training (Phase III), periodic exercise testing is the best means of providing safe and appropriate increases in exercise intensity for elderly cardiac patients. The percentage of peak heart rate used for training intensity may be increased at 6-month intervals by increments of 5%, up to a level of 85% of the attained peak heart rate on the most recent sign- or symptom-limited graded exercise test. Exercise training intensities are not generally increased beyond 85% of attained peak heart rate in the elderly patient population because of the potential for musculoskeletal injury. Table 4.1 provides examples of training heart rates and their progression from Phase II to Phase III. Recent information on the health benefits of low-intensity exercise suggests that high-intensity exercise may not be required to obtain a variety of health benefits (35). This is particularly good news for the elderly.

Frequency of Exercise

Particularly during Phase II, when low exercise training intensities are dictated by low functional capacities and musculoskeletal limitations, it is important to encourage elderly patients to adhere to off-day walking or cycling programs (200). That is, recommend informal exercise on days when they do not participate in a formal session. This exercise is essential to provide an adequate training stimulus and to increase functional capacity during the initial weeks of the program.

Table 4.1   Examples of Training Heart Rate Data for Patients Participating in Phase II and Phase III Exercise Training

	Patients not on beta blockade	Patients on beta blockade
Initial THR	92 bpm	81 bpm
End of Phase II THR	111 bpm	98 bpm
Phase III THR	128 bpm	113 bpm
(THR at 18 months of exercise training)		

Note. THR = training heart rate.
Compiled from Williams, Esterbrooks, and Sketch (275) and Williams and Sketch (280).

All participants in our long-term training program are asked whether they wish to participate in formal sessions either 2 or 3 days a week (280). For those who participate only 2 days per week, it is extremely important that they exercise on their own at least 1 additional day each week.

Exercise Duration

In general, the duration of the exercise session remains constant for elderly patients during Phase II (275). Changes in the exercise prescription during Phase II are made primarily by adjusting the exercise training intensity. However, exercise duration may have to be reduced during the initial weeks of Phase II for patients whose ability to exercise for an entire session is physically or emotionally limited. This is also true for younger patients on occasion. Patients incapable of sustaining aerobic exercise for the recommended duration (20 to 40 min) are encouraged to exercise more frequently during the day or to rest for longer periods during actual Phase II training sessions.

As elderly participants move into long-term exercise training, they are encouraged to lengthen the duration of activity (280). This is not mandatory, but many participants enjoy the opportunity to increase the duration of the exercise session. Increasing the exercise duration is particularly important for individuals who exercise at a low intensity. Lengthening the duration helps increase caloric expenditure and is associated with improvement of several risk factors, including obesity, lipid abnormalities, hypertension, and elevated blood glucose (35). It is not unusual for our patients to exercise for 40 to 60 min per session, with increases in exercise duration made slowly to allow for adaptation.

Modalities for Exercise

Elderly individuals routinely use the same modes of exercise as younger patients (275). As with younger patients, any elderly participant who has undergone open heart surgery is not eligible for intensive arm ergometry until 5 weeks after surgery, to allow for adequate healing of the sternotomy wound.

Many elderly persons have orthopedic problems that have resulted from or may be exacerbated by weight-bearing exercise. Some forms of exercise, such as jogging and other high-impact activities, can result in increased incidence of injuries. Even walking, although it appears to be an easy exercise modality, may be difficult for the elderly cardiac patient who has not walked much in the recent past or has relatively severe arthritis in the knee joints. Even seemingly innocent activities should be carefully considered in this patient group for potential adverse effects, especially when the activity requires the patient to bear his or her entire weight.

Bicycling is an excellent exercise that sustains aerobic activity while decreasing the potential deleterious effects of weight bearing on the lower extremities. However, outdoor bicycling may include potential sources of injury such as road hazards and the risk of falling (90). Stationary cycling is recommended for the less healthy patient, particularly for those whose balance, hearing, or vision is impaired.

Water exercise is also an excellent form of conditioning for the elderly, especially for the obese or physically limited patient (90). It allows the patient to become "weightless," thereby decreasing stress on the joints of the lower extremities. Water-resistant calisthenics can be a useful group activity. The resistance to movement can be adjusted by rotating the palms or changing the depth of water for activity (222). Swimming can provide an excellent aerobic training stimulus, but because swimming does not stress bone, it may not be a good weight-bearing activity for preventing osteoporosis. For the elderly, a primary risk with swimming is slipping in the pool area. Also, many persons are reluctant to swim because of a lack of skill, fear of the water, or personal modesty about swimming in groups. This may be particularly true for the elderly.

Exercise machines for cross-country skiing, stair climbing, and rowing can also be effective for cardiovascular fitness. Older patients should be closely supervised initially and allowed to become comfortable with the physical coordination that these machines require in order to avoid serious injury.

Many recreational activities such as golf, dancing, and tennis are excellent forms of exercise for elderly cardiac patients (281). Participants in a long-term exercise program should be encouraged to resume the safe activities that they enjoyed prior to myocardial infarction or surgery, even though they may be reluctant to do so. The rehabilitation staff should have a positive attitude and not be overly cautious when providing guidelines for resuming activity. Impaired coordination and osteoporosis increase the risk of injury for older participants performing some recreational activities, and modifications in these activities may be appropriate. Competitive activities such as the various racket sports can supplement an exercise prescription, although the level of play should reflect the individual's physical condition. Overexertion can lead to adverse consequences, especially when the element of competition causes one to ignore warning symptoms (90). Rhythmic calisthenics and dance exercise can provide both warm-up and sustained activity, but proper counseling is essential to avoid overuse and sudden twisting injuries. Exercises that support the body's weight with the arms, such as push-ups, should be performed with caution; they may cause an excessive rise in blood pressure and increase the work of the heart.

Though not often considered part of a regular exercise program, activities of daily living should also be used to supplement formal training sessions (90). Walking to the store, hedge trimming, painting, and gardening can contribute to improving fitness. Using the stairs can provide a valuable source of physical training.

Additional Considerations for the Exercise Prescription

The following specific points should be made regarding various components of the exercise program for elderly cardiac patients. Participants should carefully consider each of these before beginning the exercise program.

Warm-Up

Participants should do warm-up exercises and then follow a careful progression of the aerobic training portion of the program to reduce the likelihood of exercise-related adverse signs and symptoms or physical injuries (28, 90). Warm-up activities may range from basic stretching and calisthenics to more active, specific muscle warm-up with exercise equipment. A preliminary period of stretching and light activity involving the large muscle groups for 5 to 10 min is appropriate for most exercise training programs for elderly cardiac patients. Light work on a treadmill, cycle ergometer, or arm ergometer is also appropriate for a warm-up activity.

Flexibility

As a result of aging, sedentary lifestyle, and arthritis, elderly cardiac patients often exhibit decreased flexibility and thus are encouraged to regularly practice range-of-motion and flexibility exercises. Including some flexibility exercise as part of the warm-up is recommended, but most of the flexibility training program should be performed after the aerobic workout, when muscles and joints have been thoroughly warmed up. Flexibility exercise should be encouraged because increased flexibility not only reduces the likelihood of injury associated with exercise but reduces the risk of injury from activities of daily living.

Flexibility, or the range of motion, in most joints is imposed by the soft tissues, including the muscle and its fascial sheaths, the connective tissue (tendons, ligaments, and joint capsules), and the skin (83, 201). Increased activity through a complete range of motion improves flexibility. Several other factors influence flexibility (83). Gender accounts for some differences in flexibility; females are considerably more flexible than males. But the most important factor for this discussion is that from adulthood onward the greatest decreases in flexibility occur.

A number of laboratory and field techniques have been devised for assessing flexibility (132). However, the normative values associated with testing (excellent, average, poor, etc.) in most cases were developed using younger subjects and may be less meaningful for the older adult. Consequently, little emphasis should be placed on the actual classification of results. Rather, initial and follow-up tests should be performed to measure and later describe individual program effectiveness. Patients generally find the evaluations relatively simple to perform and helpful in demonstrating particular limitations (261).

Fortunately, there are methods for increasing flexibility, which become increasingly important for the elderly. Static stretching invoking the inverse myotatic reflex helps to improve flexibility, but range-of-motion exercises that use jerking, bobbing, or bouncing ("ballistic" stretching) invoke the stretch reflex, which actually opposes flexibility. Static stretching is safer than ballistic stretching because it does not impose sudden strains on the tissues. Ballistic stretching frequently causes severe muscle soreness, whereas static stretching does not usually cause soreness and, indeed, may help to relieve soreness. For more details on flexibility exercises, see Appendix A.

Cool-Down

An extended cool-down following physical activity is suggested for elderly cardiac patients because of the increased potential for postexercise hypotension, syncopal episodes, or arrhythmias during recovery (90). A cool-down also helps remove lactate from muscles that have been working beyond their anaerobic threshold (224). And the postexercise cool-down period decreases the chances that stiffness and muscle pain will develop, particularly early in a training program. Cool-down may include low-level activity on any available exercise equipment or just walking within the exercise area. Repeating the warm-up exercises following the active cool-down may also be valuable. Patients should avoid excessively hot showers after exercise and prolonged standing in hot and humid areas during the cool-down period.

Footwear and Floor Surface

The participant's exercise footwear should be evaluated with emphasis on well-fitted, comfortable, supportive shoes. Because of the potential circulatory limitations, reduced support from the surrounding muscles, and degenerative changes in bones and joints that occur with aging, proper footwear is particularly important for the elderly patient (90). If floor exercise is performed, the elderly may require exercise mats, even on carpeted surfaces, to avoid discomfort.

Thermoregulation

The thermoregulatory capacity of the elderly is not significantly different from that of younger patients, and it improves with increased aerobic capacity. At comparable fitness levels, core temperatures are similar between the elderly and younger persons during exercise. However, some medications, including beta blockers and phenothiazines, may impact thermoregulatory capacity. The use of diuretics and the increased potential for dehydration with exercise in the elderly should alert the rehabilitation staff to remind patients to drink plenty of fluids before, during, and after exercise. Loss of fluid during exercise could further reduce an already volume-dependent cardiac output. Elderly patients should also be aware of symptoms of dehydration such as thirst and dizziness (159).

In hot or humid weather, it is best to have elderly persons exercise in an air-conditioned facility or outside during the coolest part of the day. A guide to recommendations for exercise in the heat and humidity are found in Table 4.2. Generally, no precautions are necessary when the temperature is below 60 °F. Extreme caution should be used when the temperature is 85 °F or above, regardless

Table 4.2 Temperature-Humidity Index

% Relative humidity	Temperature (°F)								
	60	65	70	75	80	85	90	95	100
0									
10	59	62	64	67	69	72	74	77	79
20	59	62	65	68	70	73	76	79	82
30	59	62	65	68	72	75	78	81	84
40	59	63	66	69	73	76	79	83	86
50	59	63	67	70	74	76	81	85	88
60	60	63	67	71	75	79	83	87	91
70	60	64	68	72	76	81	85	88	93
80	60	64	69	73	78	82	86	91	95
90	60	65	69	74	79	84	88	93	98
100	60	65	70	75	80	85	90	95	100
			Caution		*Extreme caution*				

From "Outpatient Program: Community Based" by J.H. Checkett. In *Cardiac Rehabilitation: Implications for the Nurse and Other Health Professionals* (p. 258) by P.S. Fardy, J.L. Bennett, N. L. Reitz, and M.A. Williams (Eds.), 1980, St. Louis: Mosby. Copyright 1980 by C.V. Mosby Company. Reprinted by permission.

of the humidity. Whether extreme or moderate precautions should be made at temperatures between 60 °F and 84 °F depends on the humidity level.

The Impact of Medications

With few exceptions, elderly patients participating in cardiac rehabilitation are taking cardiovascular medications, many of which can alter exercise performance and physiological responses (124). Medications include those used to treat hypertension, left ventricular dysfunction and congestive heart failure, angina pectoris, and arrhythmias. Information on cardiovascular medications relative to the specific needs and limitations of the elderly is needed to interpret, prescribe, and modify exercise (124).

There may be synergistic effects of exercise, medications, and the aging process (168, 266). The physiological reasons for this and the therapeutic adjustments required when elderly cardiac patients enter into exercise training should be carefully considered by the rehabilitation staff. With advancing age, major changes occur in drug absorption, metabolism, distribution, excretion, and receptor sensitivity. Elderly patients have increased adverse responses to drug therapy because of drug interactions; diminished renal, hepatic, gastrointestinal, and central nervous function; decreased lean body mass for drug distribution; and lessened compensatory responses. They also may have decreased stroke volume and cardiac output and increased total peripheral resistance; increased systolic blood pressure and decreased diastolic blood pressure; and decreased oxygen consumption—all of which may affect drug efficacy at rest and with exertion (168).

Drug sensitivity is an important concern. Deterioration of the sympathetic nervous system with aging is partly a result of decreased beta-receptor reactivity (168). This is reflected not only in altered baroreceptor activity but also in a gradual decrease in renal function. The decrease in renal function with aging may be augmented not only by underlying hypertension but also by antihypertensive drugs that are eliminated through the kidney. In the latter instance, these medications may accumulate and produce adverse responses, including significant hypertension or bradycardia. In elderly patients with reduced renal function, high-normal or slightly elevated serum potassium concentrations may exist, a condition that may be aggravated by potassium-sparing diuretics, beta-adrenergic blocking drugs (atenolol, nadolol), angiotensin-converting enzyme (ACE) inhibitors, adrenergic inhibitors (clonidine), and nonsteroidal anti-inflammatory drugs (168). It may be further enhanced in the patient who has insulin-dependent diabetes and a degree of renal insufficiency.

Aging may also affect liver function by decreasing hepatic blood flow, caused by a reduction or redistribution of cardiac output (1). So there may be a reduction in liver metabolizing capacity and an accumulation of metabolized drugs.

Diuretic Therapy

Hypertension is a significant problem in the elderly. Our own data suggest that as many as 40% of elderly patients entering outpatient cardiac rehabilitation have a history of this disease. Diuretic therapy has been and continues to be an important choice in antihypertensive therapy (182). Diuretic medications are also used in the management of congestive heart failure.

Although the exercise prescription does not have to be altered for patients taking diuretics, several concerns relate specifically to the elderly and exercise (124). Hypotension may result from excessive fluid loss. Excessive potassium loss may produce hypokalemia and result in muscle fatigue and weakness, electrocardiogram abnormalities including ST-T wave changes, and arrhythmias (205). Digitalis toxicity may also result from hypokalemia. Other adverse effects may include elevated serum cholesterol and glucose levels and elevated serum uric acid levels that may precipitate gouty arthritis. Diuretics may adversely alter sodium and magnesium levels. The risk of dehydration during exercise is also increased. In addition to the potential for reduced cardiac output in patients with coronary heart disease, diuretic therapy can further reduce cardiac performance and worsen hypovolemia, especially in the elderly patient, and can ultimately produce hypotension and associated symptoms (168). In studies of patients receiving treatment with diuretics, the use of these medications has been associated with more frequent and severe side effects than has the use of a placebo (182).

An increase in dietary intake of potassium, which may include supplements, may be considered. Newer diuretics such as indapamide may have fewer side effects and may also be effective in hypertension treatment in the elderly (182).

Alpha Blockers

This classification of drugs possesses a variety of mechanisms for producing vasodilatation treatment for both hypertension and congestive heart failure (124, 167). The principle concern for the elderly cardiac patient is the potential of postexercise hypotension and problems that may arise in conjunction with hypovolemia (124). It is imperative that elderly patients on alpha blockers participate in active cool-down following exercise to promote venous return and to reduce the potential for hypotension.

Peripheral-acting short-term alpha blockers such as prazosin have been shown to produce orthostatic hypotension. This adverse effect is clearly augmented because of the decrement in baroreceptor reactivity associated with aging (168). However, small doses of agents of this type with sustained action (e.g., terazosin) have a slower onset of action and appear to be very effective for treating hypertension in the elderly. They have been reported to induce little or no orthostatic hypotension or reflex tachycardia compared to shorter acting agents (182).

Alpha-2 Agonists

In the elderly, the centrally acting alpha-2 agonists (e.g., clonidine, guanfacine, guanabenz, and methyldopa), which decrease sympathetic outflow, are often less tolerated and may produce central nervous system side effects such as drowsiness, dry mouth, and fatigue. Adherence to these medications is often poor, and they are less prescribed in this population.

Calcium-Channel Blockers

All of the currently approved agents (including nifedipine, nicardipine, verapamil, diltiazem, and isradipine) are effective in treating one or more problems in the elderly such as hypertension, angina pectoris, or supraventricular arrhythmias (124, 182). The dihydropyridines (nifedipine, nicardipine, and isradipine) have negative inotropic properties and cause vasodilatation. They are most useful in treating hypertension and angina. In patients with coronary heart disease, these drugs should improve exercise capacity prior to the patient's achieving an ischemic threshold (124). Dihydropyridines have limited effect on heart rate because they do not slow atrioventricular conduction. In addition to causing vasodilatation, verapamil and diltiazem also slow atrioventricular conduction and thus reduce heart rate to a small degree. The initiation, modification of dosage, or deletion of these medications may affect the exercise prescription, depending on dosage and individual response. The exercise training response, however, does not appear to be affected by these medications.

Although the cardiovascular effects of these medications (vasodilatation, negative inotropy, and reduced heart rate) vary among the drugs as a group, the side effects generally include light-headedness, reflex tachycardia due to hypotension during the postexercise period, and peripheral edema (124). Avoidance of bradycardia and heart block, especially when using diltiazem and verapamil, requires initiation of therapy at a low dose and close follow-up. Sustained-release forms of several of these agents appear to be useful for treating both systolic and diastolic hypertension in the elderly (207). In the hypovolemic patient, the use of calcium-channel blockers, as well as vasodilators and nitroglycerin, may cause orthostatic hypotension and even syncope when standing.

Beta Blockers

Beta-blocking medications are commonly prescribed for the control of hypertension, arrhythmias, and angina pectoris (124). The various classes of these drugs have similar pharmacological cardiovascular effects, although there are subtle differences in the modification of heart rate, central and peripheral responses, and respiratory and metabolic functions. In general, these agents are less effective in elderly patients (182). Although large doses can effectively reduce blood pressure in the elderly, side effects such as bradycardia, heart block, postural hypotension, drowsiness, and fatigue can be significant problems. Labetalol, pindolol, and acebutolol have produced less resting bradycardia than other beta-blocking agents and thus may be useful in selected patients.

Nonselective and selective beta-blocking medications generally reduce the heart rate response to exercise by 15 to 60 beats per min depending on the dosage, time of administration relative to exercise, and individual variability of response (124, 172). These drugs also blunt pressor responses to static as well as aerobic arm exercise. Administration of beta blockers to patients with limited exercise performance due to angina pectoris may significantly increase the exercise capacity prior to the development of symptoms (124, 193). Beta blockade should be avoided, if possible, in elderly cardiac patients who also have some degree of chronic obstructive lung disease. To prevent bronchospasm, this caution should be applied to those beta blockers with noncardioselectivity including propranolol, timolol, and nadolol.

Despite the addition of a beta blocker to an elderly cardiac patient's medical regimen, the usual relationship between the percentages of maximal heart rate and maximal oxygen uptake appears to be intact (201). So the commonly used methods of heart rate prescription (i.e., heart rate reserve and percentage of peak heart rate) can be used in these patients. Similarly, the relationship of rating of perceived exertion (RPE) to percentage of maximal oxygen uptake is not significantly altered by beta blockade (129).

Angiotensin-Converting Enzyme Inhibitors

ACE inhibitors, used clinically for over a decade, have increasingly been used to treat hypertension and congestive heart failure (CHF). As with beta blockade, they appear to be less effective in the elderly (182), but they may have specific benefit for hypertensive elderly patients with congestive heart failure. ACE inhibitors improve exercise capacity and reduce mortality rate in patients with CHF (205). They should have no effect on the exercise prescription or training (124). As with other medications that result in peripheral dilatation, precautions should be taken to avoid postexercise hypotension (167).

Nitrates

Nitrate preparations are useful for both the treatment of acute anginal episodes and the prevention of angina. The anti-anginal effects of nitrate preparations result primarily from their ability to increase coronary blood flow while reducing myocardial oxygen demand. The latter is accomplished through decreases in preload through venodilatation and in afterload through peripheral arterial vasodilatation. Although most often used to treat an acute angina episode, sublingual nitroglycerin, administered immediately before exercise, may reduce the likelihood of exertional angina, thereby enhancing exercise tolerance (124). The use of sublingual nitroglycerin may result in peripheral effects significant enough to produce hypotension and a concomitant reflex tachycardia. So the elderly should be reminded to sit as they take this medication and to report any development or exacerbation of symptoms.

The chronic use of longer acting nitrates usually results in reduced heart rate, systolic blood pressure, and rate pressure product at a given submaximal work load (167, 205, 260). This often results in improved exercise tolerance by reducing the likelihood of exertional myocardial ischemia and angina pectoris (124). Because the relationship of heart rate, RPE, and oxygen uptake is not significantly altered during the long-term administration of nitrates, the exercise prescription usually does not require alteration when nitrate therapy is initiated (205, 260).

Although effective, chronic nitrate therapy may be limited by nitrate tolerance, and this may prohibit the beneficial effects of the long-acting nitrates. Patients may, therefore, be asked to remove patches or discontinue therapy for periods during a 24-hr day to reduce this likelihood. In addition, use of chronic nitrate therapy has occasionally been associated with adverse responses, including postural hypotension with dizziness or weakness, that may require reduced dosage (124). This occurs more commonly when hypovolemia is present, as with excessive diuretic therapy or dehydration.

Digitalis

Digitalis is commonly used in the elderly for the management of congestive heart failure and atrial arrhythmias (124). Its use results in enhanced myocardial contractility and a slowing of atrioventricular conduction, both serving to improve cardiac output. So exercise tolerance is often improved in these patients. Digitalis toxicity is of concern in patients receiving diuretic drugs because of possible hypokalemia and in patients using quinidine because of arrhythmias (124). In addition, digitalis-induced ST-T wave abnormalities reduce exercise ECG test specificity in the diagnosis of ischemia.

Specific Recommendations

The following is a list of considerations that should be made in reviewing the interaction of medications and exercise in the elderly cardiac patient (168):

1. Unless necessary for angina pectoris, drugs with negative inotropic action (e.g., beta blockers and calcium blockers) should be avoided or used judiciously in patients with impaired left ventricular systolic function.
2. Because hepatic blood flow is reduced during exercise, the clearance of medications that are flow-dependent (i.e., propranolol, metoprolol, or verapamil) may be lowered and thus may produce enhanced pharmacodynamic activity during exercise.
3. Decrease in renal function during exercise may result in an enhanced pharmacodynamic effect of those medications that are eliminated through the kidneys (e.g., atenolol, nadolol, captopril, enalapril, and lisinopril).
4. Potassium retention due to reduced renal function may be augmented by both exercise and medications, as well as by diabetes mellitus. Because both dynamic and static exercise increases serum potassium, as do certain medications (including nonselective beta blockers, ACE inhibitors, and potassium-sparing diuretics), caution should be used with these various drugs. Elderly cardiac patients who have Type I diabetes with evidence of autonomic neuropathy may also have high-normal potassium. Selected medications and exercise synergistically may worsen the disease-induced increase, although in the elderly, this rise may be blunted because of reduced muscle mass due to chronic disuse. Thus, the release of potassium from skeletal muscle may not be substantial.
5. Biochemical changes induced by exercise may significantly affect the neuroendocrine system. Exercise may act as a catalyst to induce a reduction in catecholamine concentration or reactivity, or both. If sympathetic tone is elevated in the elderly cardiac patient, then a reduction in chemical mediators of the sympathetic nervous system may help explain the contribution of exercise in lowering blood pressure.

Medications and Hyperlipidemia

Hypercholesterolemia, a reduced concentration of high-density lipoprotein cholesterol, and an elevated concentration of low-density lipoprotein cholesterol have been shown to be related to development of CAD (168). Whereas changes in diet can reduce cholesterol, exercise may favorably alter the lipoprotein patterns. Drug-induced increases in low-density lipoprotein cholesterol, total cholesterol, and triglycerides by diuretics and beta blockers are probably short-term and reversible and have not been proven to worsen coronary artery or peripheral vascular disease. ACE inhibitors, calcium-channel blockers, alpha agonists, and peripheral blockers are nonlipogenic.

Specific Precautions

Elderly patients taking drugs that can cause volume depletion or orthostatic hypotension should have their blood pressure and pulse checked while lying and standing (168). Patients on diuretics need to have potassium measured periodically.

Lipid-soluble drugs, such as sedative hypnotics, tricyclic antidepressants, central alpha agonists, and beta-adrenergic blocking drugs, may alter cognitive function if given to patients who have cerebral vascular disease (168). Special care may be needed in prescribing exercise and potential lifestyle modifications for the elderly. Reinforcement of information and directions is critical. Drug therapy should be monitored and adjusted according to age and exercise-related factors that may influence drug concentration.

Resistance Training

Accidents are a major cause of injury and death in the elderly population. Many accidents can be blamed on inadequate muscle strength (253). Resistance training can help reduce these problems by promoting increases in and maintenance of acceptable levels of muscular strength and lean body mass. Increased muscle mass may also help increase maximal oxygen uptake and thus functional capacity.

Guidelines for Resistance Training

Traditional exercise guidelines for cardiac patients have emphasized aerobic activities such as walking, cycling, swimming, or jogging and have excluded resistance training because of potential adverse responses (19, 150, 166). In recent years resistive strength exercises such as weight training have gained acceptance for cardiac patients, although little attention has been placed on their value within the elderly cardiac population. Maintaining and improving strength, especially of the upper body, and developing muscle tissue should make it easier for the cardiac patient to pursue occupational or leisure-time activities. So the role of resistance training for the elderly has important ramifications for exercise program design (97, 121, 147).

Increasing muscular strength begins for most elderly cardiac patients as they begin to exercise. Strength levels are often so reduced that even the aerobic exercise program enhances strength, but further increases in strength require the addition of a resistance component. Early on in the Phase II program, patients can develop additional strength using low-weight wall pulley systems, hand-held or wrist weights, or lightweight dumbbells, as well as less quantifiable resistance devices such as elastic exercise bands. For those activities that allow for quantification of weight increments, generally 1 to 5 lb is appropriate. The patient can perform a high number of repetitions with the weights alone or can continuously use the weights while performing aerobic exercise (i.e., wear wrist weights while walking on the treadmill).

As patients develop strength, many will be interested in a more formal method of strength training. The use of greater weight loads during previously described activities will promote continued strength development. But some patients will wish to participate in a more traditional resistance-training program that uses free weights and such equipment as Universal- or Nautilus-type. Because these training modalities often use greater levels of resistance, certain precautions should be considered for evaluation, prescription, and safety.

Elderly cardiac patients should be evaluated before they participate in traditional resistance-training programs (150). They should

- have normal or normalized-controlled blood pressure,
- be free of complex arrhythmias,
- have completed 6 to 8 weeks of Phase II, and
- have at least a 5-MET functional capacity. (Some elderly patients will not be able to attain a 5-MET level of aerobic capacity. An individualized decision can be made as to whether these activities are appropriate for a patient with less functional capacity.

Patients should receive instructions in weight-training maneuvers such as how to breathe properly during these exercises and how to avoid the Valsalva maneuver. Weight training should follow aerobic conditioning in a training session. A minimum of 5 to 10 min of range-of-motion activities should be performed prior to resistance training to prepare for more vigorous activity and to prevent injury.

Resistance training must be monitored closely so that overvigorous twisting or excessive strain does not occur. Systemic blood pressure may increase more in response to anaerobic exercises such as weight training than to aerobic exercise (166). Blood pressure monitoring may be indicated in some individuals. Because of the increased risk of arrhythmias from resistance activity, electrocardiogram monitoring is recommended during the first few sessions and when increases in resistance are made. Resistance exercise has been shown to be safe, and no adverse events have been reported when patients were appropriately screened (76, 96, 163).

Circuit Weight Training

Circuit training requires the participant to exercise in short bouts, using light to moderate work loads with frequent repetitions, interspersed with short rest periods. This method of exercise challenges both the skeletal muscles and the cardiovascular system. In cardiac patients, the initial strength assessment can be performed using one repetition maximum (1RM) testing—the greatest amount of weight that can be lifted, pulled, or pushed one time for each resistance-training station. However, this testing should only be performed in individuals who have been regularly exercising using the muscle groups to be tested.

The use of 1RM testing is not recommended in persons with no recent exercise history because of the increased potential for injury and the potential of abnormal cardiovascular signs or symptoms. This concern is underscored in the elderly. If

1 RM evaluation is considered unsuitable, a method of trial and error to determine an appropriate weight load for training can be used (25). Have the patient begin with a load that is 25% of his or her body weight for larger or stronger muscle groups (e.g., quadriceps) and 10% of his or her body weight for smaller or weaker muscle groups (e.g., triceps, hamstrings). Do as many repetitions as possible with this load. All repetitions should be smoothly executed. If the patient executes 12 to 15 repetitions with this trial load, then this load is the weight to use for training. If the patient cannot perform 12 repetitions, the load is too heavy and should be lightened. If the patient can perform more than 15 repetitions, increase the work load. Use Table 4.3 to make necessary adjustments and repeat the evaluation.

Circuit training generally includes eight or fewer stations, depending upon the equipment and facilities (150). Guidelines for circuit resistance training in the elderly cardiac patient should include

1. one repetition maximum (1RM) testing,
2. a maximum of 8 to 12 repetitions,
3. resistance at 40% to 60% of 1RM,
4. 1 to 3 sets,
5. use of major muscle groups, and
6. a minimum of two training sessions per week.

Five percent increases in work load intensities up to 60% 1RM can be made following 1RM reevaluations, performed at 5- to 6-week intervals. The time for exercise at each station should be no longer than 30 s, followed by a 30- to 60-s rest period while the patient prepares for the next station. Using eight stations, with 1 set per station, would add about 12 min to the exercise training session. Even with additional stations or sets, circuit resistance training should not exceed 30 min. Longer sessions are associated with higher dropout rates, smaller

Table 4.3 Load Adjustment Chart

Repetitions completed	Adjustment (in lbs)
<7	−15
8–9	−10
10–11	−5
12–15	0
16–17	+5
18–19	+10
>20	+15

From *Weight Training: Steps to Success* (p. 114) by T.R. Baechle and B.R. Groves, 1992, Champaign, IL: Human Kinetics. Copyright 1992 by Leisure Press. Reprinted by permission.

additional gains, and perhaps the likelihood of increased injury rate. Weight-training stations that might be used in a circuit training program for the upper body include the bench press, lat pull, arm curl, and tricep pull; for the lower body, the knee extension, leg curl, leg press, and toe press could be used (25).

Strength Training

A traditional strength-training program focusing on strength alone, with little emphasis on the cardiovascular system, involves 4 to 8 repetitions at each station, with increased total work output a function of increased percentage of 1RM (60% to 80%) (25, 113). Only those elderly cardiac patients who have completed Phase II as well as a circuit training program as previously outlined should attempt strength training. For these patients, a recent echocardiogram to evaluate left ventricular function is recommended prior to initiating strength training. This evaluation may also include an echocardiogram recorded during 1RM testing to determine whether maximal resistance effort precipitates any left ventricular wall motion abnormalities.

Fewer stations are used in strength training because of the relatively high work load outputs at each station and the potential for excessive blood pressure response. Thus, one or two stations of both arm/upper torso and leg exercise are recommended. The procedure for updating work load intensities is the same as that used in the circuit training program.

Home Exercise

The staff at the Creighton University Cardiac Rehabilitation Program believe that early exercise training is best begun in a formal supervised setting (281). But because formal programs are not always available, some patients must exercise without direct supervision. The alternative of denying the benefits of exercise to a patient is unacceptable unless the person is at high risk.

Both short- and long-term exercise programs for the elderly patient for whom there is no direct supervision must be developed under specific advice from the patient's primary care physician (281). The exercise prescription can closely follow the recommendations for warm-up, flexibility, intensity, frequency, duration, modality, and cool-down outlined earlier in this chapter. However, physicians, the cardiac rehabilitation staff, and patients must take extra care to start an unsupervised exercise program cautiously. It is crucial that a patient monitor his or her own exercise response and potential cardiac symptoms and contact the primary care physician or the cardiac rehabilitation staff when any changes or symptoms occur.

Physicians and cardiac rehabilitation staff members who prescribe home exercise should also provide patients with written materials that promote compliance with the exercise prescription (281). At the Creighton Cardiac Center, for example, each patient receives a home exercise log book that outlines the basis for the specific exercise program. The exercise log book is used for recording the date, type of exercise, heart rate response, and any symptoms that may have occurred. The patient can then bring the booklet to each medical appointment or mail it to the physician or rehabilitation program for periodic review. A sample exercise log book is provided in Appendix B. Also, the American Heart Association has a series of videocassette tapes available that can assist the physician, cardiac rehabilitation staff, and patient (11). The tapes include information on both exercise and lifestyle modification.

Summary

The prescription of exercise in elderly cardiac patients should follow general guidelines used for all patients participating in cardiac rehabilitation exercise training. However, several special concerns must be considered because the elderly often have numerous concomitant limitations in addition to their cardiac status. Attainment of optimal levels of mobility, independence, and functional capacity are critical goals in this patient population. In addition to improving aerobic condition, the exercise program should provide a mechanism for enhancing flexibility, body composition, and strength in order to achieve these objectives.

Chapter 5

Training Adaptations

The objective of exercise training in elderly cardiac patients should be to limit the physical, emotional, and sociological deterioration that can result from coronary heart disease. Maintaining and improving functional capacity not only enhances mobility and personal independence but also positively affects self-image and reduces chronic anxiety and depression. Cardiac rehabilitation staff members need to understand the potential benefits of a physical activity program in this patient group so that they can help the patient understand what to expect. This chapter discusses the training adaptations of the healthy elderly and of the elderly cardiac patient.

Responses to Training in the Healthy Elderly

Exercise training responses of healthy elderly participants have received more attention (more investigations undertaken and more variables studied) than those of the elderly cardiac population. But there is no reason to suspect that, given appropriate study, healthy and cardiac elderly populations will not respond similarly. The primary differences lie in how the elderly cardiac patient can be trained and in how much time it will take to achieve similar benefits due to a more conservative approach for individuals with heart disease.

General Training Responses

The cardiovascular benefits of physical conditioning are similar in older and younger subjects, although baseline values in older subjects are lower and the elderly may require more time for adaptation (188). Maximal oxygen uptake and physical work capacity can improve as much as 40% in elderly males and females.

The amount of improvement depends on baseline values and the exercise training protocol (3, 20, 21, 38, 42, 70, 82, 87–89, 121, 187, 202, 208, 219, 229, 251). Heart rate, systolic and diastolic blood pressure, and blood lactate are reduced after training at a given submaximal work load, whereas anaerobic threshold is increased (3, 34, 47, 70, 73, 178, 188, 208, 220). Other important changes include increased oxygen pulse (the volume of oxygen consumption with each heart beat), improved cardiovascular recovery, increased duration of submaximal exertion, and lowered resting systolic and diastolic blood pressure (34, 61, 82, 84, 202, 208, 229, 244). Despite these improvements, there is no evidence that myocardial performance is altered with chronic exercise in the elderly (202). Some reports have suggested, however, that following exercise training, there is reduction in the magnitude of ST-segment depression at standardized submaximal work loads (208, 229). There is no information on the effect of training on arrhythmias in the elderly.

Peripherally, the oxidative capacity of muscle tissue increases, resulting from one or more of three factors: increased capillarization, increased aerobic enzyme content in the skeletal muscle, and preservation of the size and number of mitochondria (212, 226). Conditioning decreases body fat and increases lean mass (223, 231). Exercise can benefit carbohydrate and lipid metabolism in younger adults, and although the effects in sedentary elderly individuals are less definitive, reduced total cholesterol and low-density lipoprotein cholesterol and increased high-density lipoprotein concentrations have been reported (70, 213).

Respiration

Respiratory function does not limit exercise capacity in healthy individuals at any age. And the ventilation changes that occur with aging do not preclude significant improvement in aerobic capacity after training (99). As in younger individuals, the oxygen transport system in the elderly without respiratory disease depends more on peripheral and cardiovascular capacity than on respiratory capacity (90, 223).

Neuromuscular Function

The capacity for improved neuronal response is compromised by the progressive death of neurons with aging and an increased rigidity of response from the remaining neuron pool (90). Although an active lifestyle appears to delay the aging-related slowing of neuromuscular reaction times, there is little evidence of improved reaction time in sedentary elderly persons who have undergone a period of exercise training (240). However, the neural recruitment patterns involved in the activities that comprise the exercise program will improve.

Muscular Strength

Increases in strength from resistance training are difficult to assess. Improvement is influenced by the initial level of strength and the potential for improvement, which is affected by the presence of chronic disease. In studies of subjects aged

60 to 90, increases in strength following 6 to 26 weeks of training ranged from 9% to 227%, depending on the muscle group studied. The mean increase for all muscle groups was approximately 75% over an average of 10 weeks (12, 97, 107, 122, 149, 165, 180, 197). Strength gains in the elderly are attributed primarily to improved neural recruitment patterns and, to a lesser degree, to muscle fiber hypertrophy. In these studies, no direct correlation was noted between the degree of hypertrophy and relative strength gains (97, 107, 180); strength gains occurred within the first few weeks of training, before hypertrophy would be a factor. However, muscle hypertrophy does appear to account for some of the strength gains observed in the elderly as assessed by muscle biopsy or cross-sectional CT scanning (12, 97, 107, 160).

Resistance training may have a positive effect on blood pressure. However, results from the few studies that have investigated this hypothesis suggest either a minimal reduction of blood pressure or no effect (61, 155).

Bone Metabolism

The effects of physical activity on bone density in the elderly are not as conclusive as in younger persons, although mean bone mineral content has been observed to increase with higher intensity training in the elderly by 20% above the levels of control subjects (8, 90, 238). These few studies suggest that exercise is beneficial in increasing mineral content in the elderly who have senile osteoporosis.

Flexibility

This type of training in the elderly results in improved joint flexibility and subjective perception of improved mobility (90). A sense of well-being is also enhanced in many subjects as a result of improved flexibility, either measured or perceived (240).

Responses to Training in the Elderly Cardiac Patient

Although the results of studies have been consistent, data are sparse on the effects of exercise training in cardiac patients aged 65 or greater. Investigations have focused primarily on changes resulting from aerobic exercise performed during early postdischarge exercise rehabilitation (Phase II); fewer findings relate to the benefits of long-term aerobic exercise rehabilitation (Phase III). Clearly much work needs to be done in these areas as well as on resistance training and the psychological and sociological effects of these programs. However, results to this point strongly suggest that exercise training plays a significant role in enhancing functional capacity and enhancing lifestyle in the elderly cardiac patient.

Functional Capacity

The effects of aerobic exercise training on functional capacity can be determined by comparing pre- and posttraining exercise test results. The two principal variables compared are maximal oxygen uptake and response to submaximal effort. Examples of methods of determining changes in these responses are illustrated in Table 5.1.

In this table, changes in maximal oxygen uptake can be determined by comparing test end points, here demonstrating an increase in functional capacity of 8 METs on the pretraining test to 9 METs on the posttraining exercise test. Conversely, changes in submaximal exercise response can be determined by comparing the rate pressure product (RPP) at each level of submaximal work. Because RPP is an indicator of myocardial oxygen uptake, this example indicates a reduced myocardial oxygen uptake for each submaximal work load. The posttraining data suggest improved myocardial efficiency and reduced work of the heart for the same level of exertion. An overall change in response can be described by determining an overall mean change for the test, in this example, a mean reduction in RPP of 25%.

The use of maximal oxygen uptake, measured directly or estimated, to describe changes in functional capacity has some inherent limitations. Changes in maximal oxygen uptake between an initial test performed at the end of hospitalization or immediately after discharge and one performed after several weeks of exercise may reflect changes not specifically associated with training adaptation. For example, physicians may perform submaximal testing at hospital discharge, whereas subsequent testing may be sign- or symptom-limited maximum testing. When comparing pre- and posttraining exercise testing results, one must also consider the willingness of a physician to use maximal testing or the patient's ability to achieve a "true" maximal end point at hospital discharge testing. In addition, patients can be expected to make some spontaneous improvement over the first few weeks following hospital discharge not related to exercise training (216). Cardiac patients have also reported increases in self-confidence and less fear of physical exertion after training, with and without improvements in peripheral or cardiac measurements that allow them to exercise longer on the exercise test (33, 81, 151). Thus, although improvements following exercise training may primarily represent physiological adaptations, other factors should be considered when describing a so-called training effect.

Because of the limitations in comparing maximal oxygen uptake between exercise tests early in recovery, submaximal exercise response may be a better indicator of the benefits of exercise training. In particular, pre- and posttraining rate pressure product levels at a standardized exercise work load can be a good indicator of fitness changes. Comparisons can also be made of scores for ratings of perceived exertion obtained at each stage of submaximal exercise. It is important to compare responses at the same protocol stages when one uses this method. Comparisons are helpful in differentiating changes in response to increasing levels of exertion at low-level (2 to 4 METs), moderate (5 to 7 METs), or high-level work (greater than 7 METs). Comparisons of the angina threshold and ST-segment changes relative to myocardial oxygen consumption are also possible.

Table 5.1 Determination of Effects of Exercise Training

Work load	V̇O₂ (ml/kg)	MET	Pretraining test			Posttraining test			% change in RPP
			HR	BP	RPP (× 10²)	HR	BP	RPP (× 10²)	
2 mph at									
0% grade	7.0	2	100	120/80	120	90	110/70	99	−18
7% grade	14.0	4	115	135/80	155	100	120/70	100	−23
14% grade	21.0	6	130	150/70	195	115	120/70	138	−29
17.5% grade	24.5	7	145	170/70	247	135	130/70	176	−29
3 mph at									
12.5% grade	28.0	8	170	190/65	323	150	160/60	240	−25
15% grade	31.5	9	—	—	—	170	180/60	306	—

Note. BP = blood pressure; HR = heart rate; RPP = rate pressure product; negative sign = a decrease in the RPP. From "Principles and Methods of Exercise Testing" by M.A. Williams. In *Cardiac Rehabilitation: Implications for the Nurse and Other Health Professionals* (p. 54) by P.S. Fardy, J.L. Bennett, N.L. Reitz, and M.A. Williams (Eds.), 1980, St. Louis: Mosby. Copyright 1980 by C.V. Mosby Company. Reprinted by permission.

Participants should be evaluated after they have taken their prescribed medications. Changes in medications may affect heart rate and blood pressure response to exercise during training, making rate pressure product comparisons less valid. Circumstances that invalidate rate pressure product comparisons include commencing, discontinuing, or altering beta-blocker medications that significantly change exercise heart rate; changes in other medications that may affect either exercise heart rate or blood pressure response; and manifestations of coronary artery disease that affect the sinoatrial node and produce large differences in heart rate.

Phase II Exercise Training

Studies of the effects of up to 12 weeks of Phase II exercise training have demonstrated a variety of training benefits (4, 5, 278). Our own studies have demonstrated significantly increased maximal exercise tolerance, decreased submaximal exercise myocardial work as estimated by the rate pressure product, and decreased ratings of perceived exertion at standardized work intensities (Table 5.2). Observations of increased maximal rate pressure product after training suggest that trained elderly cardiac patients perform at higher levels of myocardial oxygen demand (278).

Other work from Ades and colleagues has demonstrated similar results (5). Our investigation and that of Ades and co-workers have demonstrated that these results are achieved regardless of whether elderly patients are taking beta blockers or are post-acute myocardial infarction or post-coronary artery bypass graft surgery patients (Tables 5.3 and 5.4). Elderly cardiac patients appear to make modest but significant improvements in weight, percentage of body fat, forced expiratory ventilation in 1 s, resting heart rate, and resting rate pressure product (Table 5.2). Resting systolic and diastolic blood pressures have not been reported to exhibit a significant training effect.

Phase III Exercise Training

In many instances, the response to long-term exercise (Phase III) is a maintenance of gains made in Phase II. Nevertheless, modest improvements have been reported in weight, resting heart rate, resting systolic blood pressure, and maximal exercise capacity (Table 5.5) (279). A significant decrease in resting diastolic blood pressure also has been observed, a finding not previously noted with short-term exercise training. Significant improvements in physiological and perceptual responses to standardized submaximal effort have also been reported and suggest continued reduction in submaximal myocardial oxygen demand at standardized work loads is possible. Improvements from short- and long-term exercise rehabilitation allow elderly patients to function at higher work levels during daily activities and may result in fewer cardiac symptoms and improved quality of life.

Males Versus Females

Although few investigators have compared training effects in elderly males and females, findings suggest similar improvements, even though the females studied

Table 5.2 Results of the Evaluation of Elderly Patients Before and After Training

	Before training	After training
Body weight (kg)	76.9 ± 12.2	75.2 ± 11.9*
Body fat (%)	22.3 ± 5.7	20.8 ± 5.4*
Vital capacity (liters) ($n = 34$)	3.6 ± 0.6	3.6 ± 0.5
FEV$_1$ (% of vital capacity) ($n = 34$)	73.9 ± 12.1	79.4 ± 7.4*
Before exercise		
HR (beats/min)	77 ± 14	68 ± 9*
Systolic BP (mmHg)	125 ± 21	122 ± 19
Diastolic BP (mmHg)	76 ± 10	73 ± 9
Maximal exercise		
HR	126 ± 20	138 ± 20*
Systolic BP	161 ± 27	171 ± 24*
HR × BP × 10^{-2}	205 ± 55	234 ± 48*
Physical work capacity (METs)	5.3 ± 1.3	8.1 ± 1.6*
Submaximal exercise		
Average HR × BP × 10^{-2}	173 ± 44	141 ± 35*
Average RPE	12 ± 2	10 ± 2*

Note. Mean values ± standard deviations. $N = 76$; $M = 70.2 ± 3.2$ years; BP = blood pressure; FEV$_1$ = forced expiratory ventilation in 1s; HR = heart rate; HR × BP = heart rate × systolic blood pressure; RPE = rating of perceived exertion.
*$p < .05$.
From "Early Exercise Training in Patients Older than Age 65 Years Compared With That in Younger Patients After Acute Myocardial Infarction or Coronary Artery Bypass Grafting" by M.A. Williams, C.M. Maresh, D.J. Esterbrooks, J.J. Harbrecht, and M.H. Sketch, Sr., 1985, *American Journal of Cardiology,* 55, p. 264. Copyright 1985 by American Journal of Cardiology. Reprinted by permission.

had nearly a 20% lower maximal oxygen uptake (7, 192, 198). Elderly female cardiac patients are less likely to be referred to cardiac rehabilitation than males, although they have similar clinical profiles, but they improve similarly to elderly male cardiac patients in acute and chronic exercise adaptation.

The Older Elderly

Results from previously described investigations suggest that through exercise training elderly cardiac patients are capable of significant increases in maximal exercise tolerance and significant decreases in submaximal exercise myocardial work as estimated by lower rate pressure product. Despite these findings, subjective and objective observations have suggested that older elderly cardiac patients, those ages 75 and older, may not improve as much as younger elderly cardiac patients following standard Phase II exercise training. In a study to determine if older elderly patients benefit from exercise training similarly to

Table 5.3   Test Results Before and After Training in Elderly Patients: Beta-Blockade Versus Non-Beta Blockade

	Before training	After training
Beta blockade ($n = 25$)		
Physical work capacity (METs)	5.1 ± 1.5	$7.8 \pm 1.4*$
Average HR $\times$ BP $\times$ 10^{-2} (submaximal)	155 ± 38	$125 \pm 28*$
Average RPE (submaximal)	13 ± 2	$11 \pm 2*$
Non-beta blockade ($n = 51$)		
Physical work capacity (METs)	5.4 ± 1.2	$8.2 \pm 1.6*$
Average HR $\times$ BP $\times$ 10^{-2} (submaximal)	$182 \pm 44†$	$149 \pm 35*†$
Average RPE (submaximal)	12 ± 2	$10 \pm 2*$

Note. Mean values ± standard deviations. HR × BP = heart rate × systolic blood pressure; RPE = rating of perceived exertion.
*$p < .05$; †Significantly different ($p < .05$) from beta-blockade group.
From "Early Exercise Training in Patients Older Than Age 65 Years Compared With That in Younger Patients After Acute Myocardial Infarction or Coronary Artery Bypass Grafting" by M.A. Williams, C.M. Maresh, D.J. Esterbrooks, J.J. Harbrecht, and M.H. Sketch, Sr., 1985, *American Journal of Cardiology*, 55, p. 265. Copyright 1985 by American Journal of Cardiology. Reprinted by permission.

Table 5.4   Test Results Before and After Training in Elderly Patients: AMI Versus CABGS

	Before training	After training
After AMI ($n = 41$)		
Physical work capacity (METs)	5.4 ± 1.3	$8.0 \pm 1.4*$
Average HR $\times$ BP $\times$ 10^{-2} (submaximal)	168 ± 43	$135 \pm 33*$
Average RPE (submaximal)	13 ± 2	$11 \pm 2*$
After CABG ($n = 35$)		
Physical work capacity (METs)	5.1 ± 1.3	$8.1 \pm 1.8*$
Average HR $\times$ BP $\times$ 10^{-2} (submaximal)	179 ± 44	$148 \pm 36*$
Average RPE (submaximal)	12 ± 2	$10 \pm 2*$

Note. Mean values ± standard deviations. AMI = acute myocardial infarction; CABGS = coronary artery bypass grafting surgery; HR × BP = heart rate × systolic blood pressure; RPE = rating of perceived exertion. *$p < .05$.
From "Early Exercise Training in Patients Older Than Age 65 Years Compared With That in Younger Patients After Acute Myocardial Infarction or Coronary Artery Bypass Grafting" by M.A. Williams, C.M. Maresh, D.J. Esterbrooks, J.J. Harbrecht, and M.H. Sketch, Sr., 1985, *American Journal of Cardiology*, 55, p. 264. Copyright 1985 by American Journal of Cardiology. Reprinted by permission.

Table 5.5   Elderly Cardiac Patient Training Response Following 18 Months of Exercise Training

	Pretraining (T_1)	After 3 months of training (T_2)	After 18 months of training (T_3)
Weight (kg)	79.5 ± 12.3	77.5 ± 11.6*	76.1 ± 12.1
% Body fat	22.8 ± 5.5	20.4 ± 4.8*	20.4 ± 4.6
Resting heart rate (bpm)	83 ± 11	77 ± 13*	73 ± 11
Resting systolic blood pressure (mmHg)	121 ± 17	120 ± 16	117 ± 15
Resting diastolic blood pressure (mmHg)	84 ± 9	77 ± 11*	69 ± 10†
Maximal heart rate (bpm)	122 ± 22	134 ± 22*	130 ± 18
Maximal systolic blood pressure (mmHg)	158 ± 27	168 ± 27*	166 ± 14
Maximal rate pressure product/100	193 ± 49	225 ± 48*	216 ± 33
Maximal exercise capacity (METs)	4.9 ± 1.7	8.1 ± 20*	8.6 ± 2.4
Submaximal average rate pressure product/100	202 ± 49	134 ± 26*	113 ± 25†
Submaximal average RPE	12 ± 2	10 ± 2*	9 ± 1†

Note. Mean values ± standard deviations. Patient age $M = 69.3 ± 2.9$; $N = 18$.
*$p < .05$ for T_1 vs. T_2; †$p < .05$ for T_2 vs. T_3.
Reprinted from Williams and Esterbrooks (273a) by courtesy of Marcel Dekker, Inc.

younger elderly, improvement occurred largely in patients ages 65 to 74, who made up the vast majority of patients studied before and after exercise training (276). Results are presented in Table 5.6. Limited improvements in submaximal and maximal responses to exercise were observed in cardiac patients ages 75 and older; fewer changes were observed in patients ages 80 and greater.

The results from a subsequent study on a larger group of elderly patients suggest that a subgroup of older elderly cardiac patients is capable of achieving training benefits similar to those observed in younger elderly patients (Table 5.7) (277). This subgroup was characterized as capable of completing an extended period of exercise training following the standard Phase II program; having a peak exercise capacity of at least 4 to 5 METs at the end of the standard Phase II program; and capable of increasing exercise training intensity throughout the entire period of early and extended exercise training.

Comparison of Training Adaptation in Young and Elderly Cardiac Patients

Comparisons of the exercise training benefits between young and elderly cardiac patients have demonstrated some interesting and important findings. We studied 361 male patients of varying ages who were referred for early exercise training following acute myocardial infarction or coronary artery bypass graft surgery

Table 5.6   Exercise Training Results for Elderly Cardiac Patients With Age Subgroups Before and Following 12 Weeks of Exercise Training

Variable	Test 1	Test 2
All subjects (N = 248) (M = 70.4 years) (53% post-MI and 47% post-CABGS)		
Resting		
Heart rate (bpm)	83 ± 5	78 ± 3*
Systolic pressure (mmHg)	124 ± 7	123 ± 7
Diastolic pressure (mmHg)	71 ± 4	71 ± 3
Submaximal exercise rate pressure product/100	144 ± 15	123 ± 12*
Maximal exercise		
Heart rate (bpm)	129 ± 7	131 ± 7
Systolic pressure (mmHg)	167 ± 9	172 ± 8*
Rate pressure product/100	215 ± 19	225 ± 16*
Functional capacity (METs)	3.2 ± .5	6.5 ± .6*
Age subgroup 1 (n = 135) (M = 66.9 years) (52% post-MI and 48% post-CABGS)		
Resting heart rate (bpm)	85 ± 7	79 ± 5*
Submaximal exercise rate pressure product/100	148 ± 22	126 ± 18*
Functional capacity (METs)	3.4 ± .7	7.0 ± .8*
Age subgroup 2 (n = 70) (M = 72.3 years) (59% post-MI and 41% post-CABGS)		
Resting heart rate (bpm)	81 ± 13	74 ± 9
Submaximal exercise rate pressure product/100	143 ± 35	120 ± 28
Functional capacity (METs)	3.2 ± 1.0	6.9 ± 1.3*
Age subgroup 3 (n = 28) (M = 76.4 years) (60% post-MI and 40% post-CABGS)		
Resting heart rate (bpm)	85 ± 22	80 ± 14
Submaximal exercise rate pressure product/100	142 ± 65	123 ± 45
Functional capacity (METs)	3.1 ± 1.0	4.9 ± 2.4
Age subgroup 4 (n = 15) (M = 81.8 years) (67% post-MI and 33% post-CABGS)		
Resting heart rate (bpm)	75 ± 21	78 ± 16
Submaximal exercise rate pressure product/100	111 ± 86	103 ± 67
Functional capacity (METs)	2.3 ± 1.1	2.8 ± 1.8

Note. Mean values ± standard deviations. MI = myocardial infarction; CABGS = coronary artery bypass graft surgery.
*Significantly different ($p < .05$).
Reprinted from Williams and Esterbrooks (273a) by courtesy of Marcel Dekker, Inc.

(278). Each patient group demonstrated greater change than might be expected from spontaneous improvement. Comparative findings between the groups demonstrated that, although absolute values were less for the elderly compared to younger patients, the magnitude of changes and the exercise training responses were similar (Table 5.8).

Ades and co-investigators have suggested that elderly cardiac patients may, in fact, make greater improvements in submaximal response to exertion than

Table 5.7   Training Response Following 6 Months of Exercise Training in the Older Elderly Cardiac Patient

	Pretraining (T_1)	After 3 months of training (T_2)	After 6 months of training (T_3)
Resting heart rate (bpm)	83 ± 17	80 ± 13	69 ± 7*
Submaximal exercise rate pressure product/100	137 ± 35	118 ± 32	77 ± 26*
Maximal oxygen uptake (METs)	3.0 ± 9	5.1 ± 1.7	6.9 ± 1.2

Note. Mean values ± standard deviations. Age ≥ 75 years; $N = 22$. *$p < .05$.
Reprinted from Williams and Esterbrooks (273a) by courtesy of Marcel Dekker, Inc.

their younger counterparts (5). A possible explanation for that finding is that regular physical activity has not been a part of elderly patients' lives for many years; hence, improvements may represent a larger percentage change when compared with baseline measurements. Our own data, however, suggest similar levels of improvement between older and younger patients—a 20% versus 17% improvement in submaximal response for older and younger patients, respectively. In addition, as suggested by Hakki and co-workers, status of left ventricular function may be more important than age in determining exercise capacity in patients with coronary artery disease (123).

No studies have compared directly the long-term benefits derived from exercise training by elderly and younger cardiac patients. Studies of long-term exercise training in younger patients have demonstrated significant benefits in anthropometric measurements and cardiovascular measures at rest and in response to submaximal and maximal exertion (95). Some of these changes have been independently observed in elderly cardiac patients (279). Whether exercise training protocols including a more intense exercise program or a longer period of training, which have been used in younger patients, would result in similar changes in the elderly cardiac patient group has yet to be determined.

Strength

Although no studies of resistance training in elderly cardiac patients have been reported, indirect evidence suggests that such programs would be of benefit. Findings suggest resistance-training programs are of significant benefit in healthy elderly individuals, and resistance training has been demonstrated to be practical and safe and to result in significant strength gains of 25% to 50% in cardiac patients (51, 113, 150, 254).

Psychological Responses

Declines in psychological function, including decreased cognitive function, decreased reaction time, and increased prevalence of psychiatric symptoms, have

Table 5.8   Exercise Test Results Before and After Training in Four Age Groups

	Before training	After training
Group I (mean age = 40 ± 4)		
Physical work capacity (MET)	6.3 ± 1.6	9.8 ± 1.6*†
Average HR × BP × 10^{-2} (submaximal)	170 ± 33	143 ± 33*
Average RPE (submaximal)	12 ± 2	9 ± 2*†
Group II (mean age = 50 ± 3)		
Physical work capacity (MET)	6.3 ± 1.3†	9.2 ± 1.4*†
Average HR × BP × 10^{-2} (submaximal)	168 ± 46	135 ± 32*
Average RPE (submaximal)	12 ± 2	10 ± 2*
Group III (mean age = 59 ± 3)		
Physical work capacity (MET)	6.0 ± 1.7	9.0 ± 1.7*†
Average HR × BP × 10^{-2} (submaximal)	156 ± 40	135 ± 37*
Average RPE (submaximal)	12 ± 2	10 ± 2*
Group IV (mean age = 70 ± 3)		
Physical work capacity (MET)	5.3 ± 1.3	8.1 ± 1.5*
Average HR × BP × 10^{-2} (submaximal)	173 ± 44	141 ± 35*
Average RPE (submaximal)	12 ± 2	10 ± 2*

Note. Mean values ± standard deviations. HR × BP = heart rate × systolic blood pressure; RPE = rating of perceived exertion.

*Significantly different from before training value ($p < .05$).

†Absolute value is significantly different from similar value in Group IV ($p < .05$), although magnitudes of change are not significantly different with the exception of METs in Group I versus METs in Group IV.

From "Early Exercise Training in Patients Older Than Age 65 Years Compared With That in Younger Patients After Acute Myocardial Infarction or Coronary Artery Bypass Grafting" by M.A. Williams, C.M. Maresh, D.J. Esterbrooks, J.J. Harbrecht, and M.H. Sketch, Sr., 1985, *American Journal of Cardiology*, 55, p. 265. Copyright 1985 by the American Journal of Cardiology. Reprinted by permission.

been found in older adults (46, 52, 133, 203). Traditional tests of cognitive function show age-related impairments in the acquisition and manipulation of unfamiliar material and declines in some forms of memory performance (45, 69). Mood disturbances are also prevalent (199).

Several studies of younger and middle-aged subjects have shown that aerobic exercise may improve mood and may improve performance on various cognitive tasks (43, 72, 92, 102, 103, 117). Cognitive impairment is increasingly recognized as a significant problem among coronary patients, especially elderly patients (27). The relative physical fitness level of subjects also affects cognitive performance (94). In general, physically fit individuals can perform cognitive tasks better than those who are less fit. Older fit individuals perform similarly to less fit college-age individuals on reaction time (120, 243, 263). More recently, these observations, as well as reports of reduced levels of depression and anxiety and decreases in perception of chronic pain, have been described in the elderly, although methodological problems and inconsistent results have made it difficult to draw any firm conclusions (30, 39, 41, 86, 104, 177, 204, 245, 252). Despite the absence of data to suggest significant psychological improvement, subjects undergoing exercise training perceive themselves as changing on a number of important psychological, social, and physical dimensions (223, 227). Subjects felt that they were in better health and looked better. They reported improved energy level, endurance, flexibility, and sleep. Socially, subjects reported improved family and sexual relations, less loneliness, and better social lives. Psychologically, subjects reported heightened self-confidence and life satisfaction, better memory, and improved concentration.

Advocates of exercise in cardiac rehabilitation note that physical activity significantly contributes to an enhanced sense of well-being and improved mood, cognitive functioning, and behavioral adaptations (37, 94). Exercise has been associated with reduced negative emotional states (i.e., reduced anxiety, depression, and anger). There are also reports of reduced tension, fatigue, depression, and confusion, as well as greater vigor (43, 164). Other studies show that improvements in mood are most likely to be observed among those individuals who are either most physically deconditioned or most emotionally distressed at the outset of the exercise program (102, 179, 234). The elderly cardiac patient may be a member of either of these groups. But even if this is not the case, these considerations are an important aspect of exercise training in the elderly. Unfortunately, studies that have assessed changes in psychological functioning among patients with coronary heart disease show relatively few consistent improvements (39, 204). This may be because most patients do not display significant psychological dysfunction before joining an exercise program (36, 40, 130). In addition, virtually all published studies in this area have excluded older cardiac patients, which may reflect the overall cautious attitude toward exercise for the elderly by the medical community. As exercise becomes a more accepted therapeutic regimen for older cardiac patients, it will be important to assess the psychosocial benefits in greater detail (94).

Summary

Exercise training in the rehabilitation of the elderly cardiac patient increases functional capacity and enhances personal independence by decreasing the need for assistance in activities of daily life. Moreover, the sense of isolation and depression that often accompanies reduced mobility may be averted or offset by the physical improvements associated with exercise training. Exercise training is also associated with improved feelings of well-being and self-esteem. And epidemiological and laboratory studies have demonstrated that exercise conditioning favorably alters coronary heart disease risk factors. Well-designed, individualized exercise training programs that fit the elderly patient's lifestyle optimize compliance to training. However, providing the elderly cardiac patient with an exercise prescription without any support or reinforcement results in low compliance. Prudent cardiac rehabilitation policy suggests that exercise training include strategies for supervision and follow-up (159).

Chapter 6

Characteristics of Participants in Outpatient Exercise Training

As noted in chapter 1, the population of the United States at the end of this century will include a much higher percentage of elderly individuals, many of whom will have coronary heart disease (CHD). Because of the growing elderly population, and because of the documented benefits of exercise in this group, the number of elderly patients participating in cardiac rehabilitation has dramatically increased in the last 3 years. Elderly cardiac patients comprise a majority of the participants in some programs (5, 79, 282). Unfortunately, little information is available on the physical, physiological, psychological, lifestyle, and risk factor characteristics of these patients as they enter cardiac rehabilitation. As the number of participants aged 65 or greater increases, rehabilitation professionals will need to look at the characteristics of this group to determine if changes are necessary in our cardiac rehabilitation programs. This chapter describes some of the characteristics of the elderly population as a whole as well as those of elderly patients entering cardiac rehabilitation exercise training programs.

Risk Factors

Group data describing medical history, indication for rehabilitation, and present medical condition (including medications, exercise capacity, and risk factor profile) have generally not been reported for elderly patients entering outpatient cardiac rehabilitation. The Framingham Heart Study and other studies have provided risk factor data for the elderly, including prevalence of hypertension, hypercholesterolemia, cigarette smoking, diabetes mellitus, glucose intolerance, and obesity (14, 145). These data, though helpful, may be limited in that they often describe the elderly population as a whole rather than the specific elderly cardiac population entering cardiac rehabilitation. Analysis of data that specifically describe the elderly cardiac patient population as it enters rehabilitation is important in order to provide appropriate patient management strategies for this particular group (which will be addressed in chapter 7). Unfortunately, risk modification as a means to lower morbidity or mortality has received less attention in elderly patients with diagnosed coronary heart disease than in the elderly population as a whole. Nonetheless, these reports can be helpful in describing the prevalence of risk factors and future risk of events in elderly cardiac patients.

Hypertension

The mechanisms of hypertension in the elderly are similar to those in younger individuals. Increased peripheral vascular resistance (PVR) plays a major role. Both mean arterial pressure and PVR increase with advancing age. Atherosclerotic and calcific changes in the aorta and other arteries reduce compliance and contribute to systolic hypertension, whereas increased PVR leads to the diastolic hypertension seen in the elderly (169).

The Framingham data suggest that systolic hypertension (>160 mmHg) is a significant risk factor for CHD in elderly males and females, whereas diastolic hypertension (>95 mmHg) is a significant risk factor only in females (145). In people ages 65 to 85, the prevalence of hypertension is 20% to 46% in men and 48% to 65% in women. Prevalence increases with age. In contrast, Aronow et al. have suggested that hypertension is significantly correlated with coronary disease in elderly women but not in elderly men (17). Compared to the Framingham data, Aronow et al. observed a similar prevalence of hypertension for elderly men (29%) but a lower prevalence for elderly women (37%) (17). They also demonstrated that hypertension in elderly subjects with previously documented CAD correlated with new coronary events (14). Demographic differences between the two study populations may explain the differences in prevalence data. Data from Aronow et al. were obtained from a long-term health care center with generally older patients, whereas the Framingham data represent individuals from a community setting (Framingham, MA) of a cross-sectional age range among the elderly. Thus, the Aronow et al. data suggest that persons who have lived longer might be expected to have a lower prevalence of hypertension because those who are hypertensive die earlier in life from cardiovascular disease.

Hypertension should be treated in the post-myocardial infarction patient even though early data suggested that low blood pressure following myocardial infarction predicts a poor prognosis (66). These observations probably reflected the degree of myocardial damage associated with extensive myocardial infarction. Analysis of patients with preexisting hypertension or those developing hypertension post-myocardial infarction indicates a greater risk of mortality, recurrent myocardial infarction, and stroke compared to those without hypertension (60). Treatment clearly reduces this risk (134).

Hyperlipidemia

Hypercholesterolemia is a primary risk factor in the elderly (13, 14, 16, 17, 29, 55, 106, 211, 232, 241, 283). From guidelines developed for younger individuals, it is clear that significant lipid abnormalities are common even in the elderly (15). Elevated serum total cholesterol (CHOL), lowered levels of high-density lipoprotein cholesterol (HDL-C), and elevated CHOL/HDL-C ratio have all been shown to be significant risk factors for mortality from CHD in the elderly and predictive of new coronary events in elderly men and women with CAD (14, 29, 145). Additionally, recent analysis revealed that among patients with prior myocardial infarction, elevated serum total cholesterol was most strongly related to increased rate of death from coronary disease and to all-cause mortality in persons aged 65 or greater (283). However, specific criteria for abnormal lipid levels in the elderly have yet to be established.

Findings suggest that 9% to 17% of elderly men and 18% to 40% of elderly women have cholesterol levels in excess of 250 mg/dl (14, 145). Whether preventive measures such as dietary modification or drugs that decrease serum total cholesterol levels while increasing or maintaining HDL-C levels have an important impact on CHD in the elderly remains to be demonstrated. Results from a few studies are favorable (53, 74, 241).

In the Framingham Heart Study, an elevated serum triglyceride level was found to be a significant risk factor for CAD in elderly women but not in men (55). Aronow et al. reported that elevated serum triglyceride level was an independent risk factor for new coronary events in both elderly men and women, with and without prior CHD events (14). In the Stockholm Ischemic Heart Disease Study, there was a significant decrease in mortality of 28% in patients over age 60 who were treated medically to reduce triglyceride level compared to untreated patients (53). Participants in this study were less than 4 months post–myocardial infarction, and approximately 50% were 65 years of age or greater. Hypertriglyceridemia occurred in 50% of the patients, whereas hypercholesterolemia was present in only 13%. A 36% decrease in CHD mortality was related to a reduction in serum triglyceride.

Smoking

Thirty-year follow-up data from the Framingham Heart Study in persons who reached age 65 or greater demonstrated that smoking was not significantly associated with total CAD incidence in the elderly but was a significant factor for cardiac death (145). The prevalence of smokers in the elderly population ranges from 9% to 22% for men and 3% to 23% for women, although there are few data for elderly women (14, 145). Smoking has been significantly correlated with new coronary events in elderly persons who have CAD (14).

Smoking cessation lowers the risk of death or myocardial infarction similarly in young and elderly patients with CAD (131, 142). In patients aged 65 or greater with documented CAD, 6-year follow-up data show that continuation of a smoking habit was associated with an 18% increase in death or myocardial infarction compared to those patients who had quit smoking (131).

Also, considerable inferential data suggest a beneficial effect of smoking cessation for the elderly cardiac patient. In the Coronary Drug Project, patients who continued smoking after myocardial infarction had a 29% higher mortality at 5 years than did those who quit smoking (65). The Framingham data demonstrated fewer recurrent myocardial infarctions and reduced mortality in those who stopped smoking (242). Other work has resulted in similar findings (270). Although these data are not specific to the elderly, the mean population age at follow-up was greater than 60 in most studies.

Cigarette smoking is also strongly related to several other diseases, including emphysema and lung cancer. So in addition to the association of smoking with CHD risk in the elderly, there are other reasons why smoking cessation is a health measure that should be strongly encouraged in this group.

Diabetes Mellitus

Diabetes mellitus and glucose intolerance represent extremely potent risk factors for cardiovascular and coronary mortality in the elderly, especially in women. From the Framingham data, the prevalence of glucose intolerance is 29% to 34% in men and 17% to 29% in women (145). Aronow et al. observed a lower prevalence for men (14%) and a similar prevalence for elderly women (20%) (14). Aronow et al. also demonstrated a significant correlation between diabetes mellitus and new coronary events in patients with CAD.

Presumably, the microvascular disease that is unique to diabetes, as well as other mechanisms, produces progressive damage to heart muscle and results ultimately in compromised ventricular function and heart failure. However, there is little evidence that control of hyperglycemia, either by oral hypoglycemic agents or insulin, effectively forestalls the development of complications of cardiovascular disease, especially mortality. Present evidence suggests that it is crucial to reduce the risks of CHD in elderly patients with diabetes by correcting associated risk factors.

In addition to the well-documented association of diabetes mellitus with CHD, epidemiological data suggest that hyperinsulinemia is itself an independent risk factor for cardiovascular disease (246). Limited evidence suggests that insulin may promote the growth of vascular cells and atherosclerosis. Insulin resistance has also been implicated in the pathogenesis of essential hypertension and hypertriglyceridemia (206). The term *syndrome X* has been applied to the clinical association of insulin resistance, hypertension, and increased very low density lipoprotein (VLDL) and decreased HDL-C concentrations in plasma.

Obesity

Early reports evaluating the impact of body weight on the development of cardiovascular disease failed to demonstrate an independent and significant role for obesity in the elderly. The level of risk was variable when other risk factors were taken into account. This led to the prevailing notion that being overweight exacerbated risk primarily through its relationship with other risk factors more directly related to the development of atherosclerosis, especially hypertension, hypercholesterolemia, and hyperglycemia. More recent information, however, has modified this belief. Follow-up from the Framingham cohort clearly documents a strong and independent contribution of body weight to the development of cardiovascular disease, including CHD, even when other risk factors are taken into account (145). Aronow et al. reported the prevalence of obesity in the elderly as being relatively low, approximately 5%, but did demonstrate a significant correlation between obesity and new coronary events in elderly females with CAD (14). These findings emphasize the importance of maintaining ideal body weight in elderly cardiac patients.

Descriptive Characteristics and Risk Factors in Elderly Cardiac Rehabilitation Outpatients

Unfortunately, few data describe the elderly cardiac patient population entering outpatient exercise training programs. This section describes the profile of elderly cardiac patients entering the program at the Creighton University Cardiac Center by several variables: gender; medical indication for Phase II rehabilitation; expected employment status; smoking history; prevalence of elevated cholesterol, hypertension, diabetes mellitus, and obesity; history of complex ventricular arrhythmias; poor exercise capacity at program entrance; and prevalence of exercise-induced myocardial ischemia. The data, which were compiled for elderly subjects who entered Phase II cardiac rehabilitation within 4 weeks of their most recent hospitalizations between 1981 and 1992, are summarized in Table 6.1. The data for elderly participants are compared to similar data collected for younger participants in our exercise training program.

Table 6.1 indicates that, compared to younger patients, the elderly group had a significantly greater percentage of patients whose indication for Phase II cardiac rehabilitation was recent coronary artery bypass graft surgery (CABGS) (48% vs. 33%) ($P < .05$) and a significantly lower percentage whose indication was recent percutaneous transluminal coronary angioplasty (PTCA) (3% vs. 11%). Significantly fewer elderly patients expected to be working following recovery (19% vs. 86% in the younger patient group), and the elderly patient group had significantly fewer smokers at the time of hospitalization (17% vs. 50%). Compared to younger patients, the elderly patient group had significantly greater percentages of individuals with hypertension (41% vs. 21%), poor exercise capacity (41% vs. 32%), and history of complex ventricular arrhythmias (28% vs. 20%). None of the remaining variables differed significantly between groups.

Comparison of data describing elderly patients in our outpatient exercise program to those from other studies suggests similar incidences of hypertension, hypercholesterolemia, and cigarette smoking (Table 6.2). The incidence of diabetes mellitus in our elderly cardiac patients was somewhat lower than that

Table 6.1   Comparison Data for Elderly Versus Younger Patient Groups

Variable	Group I (N = 191)	Group II (N = 414)
Sex		
Males (%)	92	86
Females (%)	8	14
Indication for Phase II		
Myocardial infarction (%)	42	46
Coronary artery bypass graft surgery (%)	48*	33
Valve replacement (%)	3	2
Percutaneous transluminal coronary angioplasty (%)	3*	11
Medical management (%)	3	8
Expected employment status	19*	86
Smoking history	17*	50
Cholesterol (% greater than 240 mg/dl)	18	23
Hypertension (%)	41*	21
Diabetes (%)	17	18
Obesity (%)	42	36
Complex ventricular arrhythmias (%)	28*	20
Peak oxygen uptake (% 3 MET or less)	41*	32
Exercise-induced myocardial ischemia (%)	25	25

Note. Patients in Group I were 65 years of age or older; patients in Group II were younger than 65.

*Significantly different from younger group ($p < .05$).

Compiled from Williams (272).

described from the Framingham data but similar to that reported by Aronow et al. (14, 145). Obesity was much more prevalent in our elderly cardiac patients compared to those of Aronow et al. but was in the range reported for the Framingham data.

Special Populations Within the Elderly

Many elderly cardiac patients have one or more chronic diseases that can affect both responses to exercise testing and the exercise prescription. Therefore, exercise testing and exercise prescription methods must be flexible and modifiable for these patients. Modifying the testing procedures allows for appropriate measurement of functional capacity and cardiovascular response to exertion. Modifying the exercise prescription permits elderly cardiac patients with a wide range of functional limitations to begin an exercise training program and to benefit. The balance of this chapter complements the information presented in chapters

Table 6.2 Prevalences of Selected Risk Factors in the Elderly

	Framingham (145)		New York City (14)		Omaha (272)	
Hypertension						
Males	20%–46%	> 160/95 mmHg	29%	> 160/90 mmHg	41%	> 140/90 mmHg
Females	48%–65%		37%		—	
Elevated total cholesterol (T-chol)						
Males	9%–17%	> 250 mg/dl	9%	≥ 250 mg/dl	23%	> 240 mg/dl
Females	18%–40%		24%		—	
High-density lipoprotein (HDL)						
Males	—		24%	< 35 mg/dl	28%	< 40 mg/dl
Females	—		15%		—	
Elevated T-chol/HDL						
Males	—		12%	≥ 6.5	45%	> 4.95
Females	—		12%		—	
Elevated triglyceride level						
Males	—		13%	≥ 190 mg/dl	32%	> 160 mg/dl
Females	—		18%		—	
Smoking						
Males	9%–22%		12%		17%	
Females	3%–23%		4%		—	
Glucose intolerance						
Males	29%–34%	> 120 mg/dl	14%	diabetes	17%	> 115 mg/dl
Females	17%–29%		20%		—	
Obesity						
Males	7%–53%	> 20% above ideal weight	4%	≥ 20% above ideal weight	42%	> 18% body fat
Females	30%–48%		6%		—	

3 and 4 on exercise testing and prescription by describing considerations in various elderly patient subgroups.

Patients With Pacemakers

We estimate that 5% of our elderly patients within the Creighton University Cardiac Rehabilitation Program have an implanted pacemaker. Permanent pacemakers are used to manage cardiac electrical conduction or rhythm disturbances. Exercise testing in patients with pacemakers is performed for several reasons unique to these patients, including the evaluation of pacemaker function and pacer programming or reprogramming, as well as for those indications for the elderly cardiac patient described in chapter 3. Graded exercise testing in patients with permanent pacemakers requires an understanding of the patient's medical status and the type and specific programming parameters of the pacemaker.

Throughout the graded exercise test, standard patient observation and recording procedures should be used, and electrocardiogram rhythm strips documenting changes in pacer function and paced complex morphology should be recorded as necessary (205). Because the ST segment may not reflect ischemic changes, exercise testing for the evaluation of CAD should include other modalities such as radionuclide or echocardiographic imaging. Depending on the type of pacemaker and its programmed characteristics, the normal linear relationship of heart rate and systolic blood pressure to increasing exercise intensity may not be present. Patients with pacemakers can demonstrate accelerated, depressed, or nonlinear ventricular rate responses to increasing exercise intensity. Systolic blood pressure may rise, plateau, or fall during activity and must be analyzed in conjunction with the patient's clinical history, symptoms, and pacemaker function. As with elderly patients in general, patients with pacemakers are likely to have low functional capacities. Thus, reduced initial work loads and incremental increases are recommended for graded exercise testing.

The exercise prescription should be carefully designed with respect to intensity, frequency, duration, and modality (196). Certain pacemakers may limit exercise. Exercise prescriptions for patients with pacemakers should be based on exercise test results whenever possible (205). Because of the potential limitation in heart rate response previously described, the use of standard exercise heart rate formulas for prescribing exercise intensity are often inappropriate. In these cases, an estimation of activity levels using target MET level and RPE appear to be most beneficial in setting activity guidelines. If an accurate functional assessment is critical, the patient should undergo direct assessment of oxygen uptake during exercise.

In general, patients with pacemakers should be able to use all exercise modalities available in the standard cardiac rehabilitation exercise program, including upper body exercise. Specific limitations in the exercise prescription will depend on the patient's clinical history and pacemaker function (205). Patients should clearly understand their specific limitations and their pacemaker function in order to provide for safe activity and reduce their anxiety about exercise.

Patients With Automatic Implantable Cardiac Defibrillators

Patients with automatic implantable cardiac defibrillators (AICDs) are appropriate candidates for cardiac rehabilitation exercise programs. However, both the patient and the exercise supervisory personnel should clearly understand the AICD and its threshold rate for discharge. Until the likelihood of inappropriate discharge has been ruled out, both patients and staff may benefit from programs that are telemetry-monitored and directly supervised by medical professionals familiar with this technology (64). Beyond the typical exercise training benefits afforded all patients, these patients in particular will also gain significant emotional support at a critical time following AICD implantation (23). The exercise heart rate during both testing and training should have a maximal limit of 15 to 20 beats below the threshold level for the device.

Patients With Chronic Congestive Heart Failure

Elderly patients with chronic congestive heart failure (CHF) usually have limited exercise capacity as a result of ventricular dysfunction, restricted cardiac output, and sedentary lifestyles (205). In addition to the increased peripheral resistance observed in many elderly patients, a reduction in stroke volume reserve during upright exercise impairs cardiac output.

Exercise testing prior to entering exercise training is strongly recommended for the elderly patient with chronic CHF. However, despite the advantages mentioned in chapter 3, the use of protocols to estimate peak oxygen uptake may be of less value because of wide variation of responses in these patients, which may include, occasionally, good exercise capacity. Direct measurement of oxygen uptake using mild increases in exercise work loads is helpful in describing the true limitations in exercise capacity.

Patients with chronic CHF often become dyspneic and fatigued, even with modest intensity exercise (250, 259). But data demonstrate that exercise training can significantly improve functional capacity and myocardial work at standardized submaximal exercise work loads in some patients. This is primarily due to peripheral adaptation of trained muscles to enable increased oxygen extraction; little or no direct improvement in cardiac function can be expected. Interestingly, there does not appear to be a relationship between resting left ventricular function and the ability to invoke a training response; that is, even those patients with significant left ventricular dysfunction at rest may be able to achieve the expected benefit of exercise training (18, 250). Some patients also show increased maximal cardiac output due to an ability to increase maximal heart rate. These observations emphasize the important role of peripheral adaptations.

At the time they are considered for referral, CHF patients generally should have a left ventricular ejection fraction at rest greater than 20%. However, lower values are not an absolute contraindication for participation in the exercise program. In addition, because they suggest a poorer prognosis, the presence of exercise-induced ischemia and arrhythmias in these patients should be carefully considered prior to program entrance.

Because patients with chronic CHF may have a relatively poor tolerance to physical activity, several modifications are recommended in the standard exercise prescription (124). Warm-up and cool-down periods should be prolonged. Patients should be frequently reminded to limit food intake before exercise to reduce blood flow to the digestive tract. Exercise intensity should be reduced, and frequency, and subsequently duration, should be increased (171). Exercise training programs for these patients should begin at a modest intensity (40% to 60% of maximal oxygen uptake or 60% to 70% of peak heart rate if oxygen uptake data is unavailable (205). Initially, a 5- to 10-min exercise session each day may be all that is attainable (267). RPE ratings of 12 to 14 (on the 6-to-20 scale) can be a useful guide, especially when heart rate response is impaired. As patients adapt to exercise, training intensity and duration should be gradually increased in accordance with the response to exercise and the severity of the heart failure.

Increased electrocardiogram (ECG) monitoring is suggested for this group of patients because of the increased potential for serious arrhythmias (62). Blood pressure response during exercise should be serially evaluated during the first few sessions to identify patients with hypotensive responses during and after exercise. The potential for exercise to aggravate CHF is always present. Patients who show intolerance to exercise training or who require frequent adjustments in medication are poor candidates for an exercise program and should be reevaluated (205).

Patients With Pulmonary Disease

When present along with cardiac disease, chronic obstructive pulmonary diseases (COPDs)—including emphysema, chronic bronchitis, and reactive airways disease (asthma)—often result in severely limited exercise capacity in elderly patients. All patients with moderate or severe COPD should be evaluated with complete pulmonary testing prior to exercise testing.

Abnormal pulmonary function that affects ventilation and gas exchange usually results in dyspnea upon exertion and limited exercise capacity. Although exercise testing may be of limited diagnostic value for CAD in these patients, valuable information can be gained from an exercise test. In addition to the general indications for this procedure, exercise testing may aid in the evaluation of these patients by defining nonpulmonary causes for symptoms and exercise limitations, determining the necessity for oxygen therapy during exercise, and determining the level of occupation-related impairment (205).

Standard exercise test methodology for elderly cardiac patients is used, but pulmonary function monitoring in conjunction with standard cardiovascular monitoring is recommended. Ventilation assessed by monitoring breathing frequency and tidal volume; measurements of oxygen uptake, carbon dioxide production, and arterial oxygen saturation; and arterial blood gas analysis are important in these patients (205).

Most elderly cardiac patients with COPD can participate in the exercise training program; the program is inappropriate only for those patients with severe respiratory disease. The presence of pulmonary disease, however, often results in a modified approach to exercise training prescription. Attempts to reach an expected training threshold often induce dyspnea and tachypnea. Optimizing the medical treatment program, including administering oxygen during the first few weeks, may improve or prevent dyspnea and increase the elderly patient's confidence in the exercise program. The exercise prescription for the dyspneic patient should be kept at a level that minimizes breathlessness and bronchospasm (222). The exercise prescription must be individualized according to both the patient's cardiac and pulmonary statuses (205).

For most patients with COPD, physical activity has not been a regular part of their lifestyles for many years. The chronic symptoms associated with this disease, particularly when physical activity is undertaken, often result in very negative attitudes about exercise. So the rehabilitation staff should place extra emphasis on finding modalities for exercise that are as enjoyable as possible to the patient as well as those that will affect the patient's ability to perform daily activities. Provided the patient enjoys these activities, walking and stationary cycling are appropriate modes of exercise. Upper body exercises such as arm cranking or rowing may be less desirable for both the patient and the rehabilitation staff because of the potential higher ventilation required at a given work load (205). However, if patients know the possible limitations of arm exercise, they may better understand how arm exercise can be part of the exercise regimen.

Modifications in the frequency and duration of exercise may be necessary (205). Some patients may be able to exercise for only 1 or 2 min before requiring rest. Short-duration exercise may be necessary until adaptations are made that enable the patient to increase the work intervals. RPE may provide patients with a supplementary or alternative monitoring procedure because very high heart rates may be observed with minimal exercise. Bottom line: Do what is tolerable.

For a patient with both cardiac and pulmonary disease, realistic expectations about chronic exercise should be based on the patient's clear understanding of both diseases, alone and in combination (205). Although these patients do not exhibit improvements in pulmonary function, COPD patients may increase exercise tolerance due to peripheral adaptation to exercise training. So symptoms related to the pulmonary disease process such as shortness of breath and anxiety related to exertion may improve, and the patient may gain an increased ability to perform activities of daily living. Also, depression resulting in an inability to function normally may improve as patients become more active.

Patients With Hypertension

Standard exercise testing methods and protocols may be used to evaluate patients with hypertension (205). The major limitation in standard testing, however, is the increased potential for uninterpretable ST segments in the exercise electrocardiograms due to the high prevalence of left ventricular hypertrophy. Even though flat or downward depression of 2 mm or greater from the resting level is suggestive of myocardial ischemia, additional exercise evaluation modalities including radionuclide and echocardiographic imaging may be needed in the diagnosis of coronary artery disease (237).

The recommended frequency for exercise training in the hypertensive patient should be similar to that employed in the elderly cardiac patient exercise program (205). High-intensity exercise should be discouraged. Resistance training is not absolutely contraindicated in hypertensive patients provided the guidelines presented in chapter 4 for this form of training are employed.

Patients With Peripheral Vascular Disease

Peripheral vascular disease (PVD) is especially common in the elderly and is frequently associated with CAD (185, 205). Elderly cardiac patients with PVD typically experience ischemic pain (claudication) in the muscles of the lower leg. The discomfort is frequently described as a tightness or cramping sensation during actual physical activity that disappears upon cessation of the exercise.

Standard exercise test methodology employed for the elderly cardiac patient can also be used in this group (205). Additional data collected during testing should include subjective ratings of pain severity associated with the PVD (Table 6.3). Testing for the evaluation of CHD should use muscle groups not limited by PVD. Peripheral discomfort associated with exertion is the primary limitation of most elderly patients with PVD during treadmill exercise, and bicycle or arm ergometry testing can be a useful alternative for some individuals. Pharmacological stress testing protocols with myocardial perfusion or left ventricular function imaging are also frequently used to evaluate these patients.

The amount of exercise that provokes symptoms varies, but exercise tolerance can be significantly limited. However, exercise training in patients with PVD often results in increased symptom-limited functional capacity. Reasons for this improvement may include one or more of the following: collateral vessel formation, improved distribution of blood flow, microvascular changes in the muscle, and improved oxidative capacity in the muscle (205). Thus, activity using the

Table 6.3   Scale for Rating of Pain or Discomfort Associated With Peripheral Vascular Disease

Rating	Description of intensity of discomfort
Grade I	Minimal discomfort or pain
Grade II	Moderate discomfort or pain, but not limiting
Grade III	Intense discomfort or pain that limits exercise
Grade IV	Excrutiating discomfort or pain resulting in immediate cessation of exercise

From *Guidelines for Exercise Testing and Prescription* (4th ed.) (p. 73) by the Preventive and Rehabilitative Exercise Committee, American College of Sports Medicine, 1991, Philadelphia: Lea & Febiger. Copyright 1991 by Lea & Febiger. Adapted by permission.

muscles affected by the disease at an intensity less than that which provokes significant discomfort is recommended. Using other modalities for exercise of nondiseased muscle groups is also recommended to augment the exercise program.

Exercise should be performed daily at an intensity that elicits tolerable discomfort, with intermittent rest periods. Patients should start with 10 to 20 min of interval exercise twice daily and, within the first few weeks of training, increase the total time of the exercise to the standard recommendations for exercise duration. As functional capacity improves, cardiac limitations may assume greater significance related to exercise limitations.

Patients With Diabetes Mellitus

Guidelines for both exercise testing and exercise prescription for patients with diabetes are similar to those for healthy adults (205). However, the response to exercise in the elderly cardiac patient who also has insulin-dependent diabetes depends on several factors: levels of exogenous insulin, the patient's knowledge of and compliance to insulin and dietary requirements, the patient's understanding of symptoms associated with hypoglycemia, and the patient's and the rehabilitation staff's knowledge and understanding of the interaction of diabetes and CAD—including the increased prevalence of silent myocardial ischemia in these patients (262).

Early in the program, exercise intensity should be maintained near the low end of the functional capacity exercise prescription range. Although the intensity may be prescribed by heart rate, for those with autonomic neuropathy and chronotropic incompetency, intensity may best be prescribed using RPE. Whenever possible, the frequency of exercise should be daily so that a regular pattern of insulin dosage (if required), diet, and caloric expenditure can be managed to maintain appropriate glucose control and to aid in weight control.

Although Type I diabetes must be under adequate control before the patient begins an exercise program, this is not to suggest that the patient will be free of problems during the program. Patients with diabetes may need periodic evaluation of the metabolic control of the disease; the risk of hypoglycemia is of particular concern (168). Blood glucose monitoring before and after exercise to determine the effect of physical activity should be an integral part of the diabetic patient's exercise routine, particularly when he or she is beginning an exercise program or when changes in the exercise prescription are made. To reduce the potential for exercise-related hypoglycemia, the patient may need to reduce insulin dosage or increase carbohydrate intake prior to exercising. Insulin adjustment or dietary changes must be performed only under direction of the patient's physician. Regardless of whether changes have been made, periodic monitoring on at least a monthly basis is valuable. For patients undergoing blood sugar analysis prior to exercise, upper limits should be established by the physician for participation in exercise. In no case should the patient be allowed to exercise when the blood sugar is in excess of 250 mg/dl.

Hypoglycemia is reported to be relatively common in patients with diabetes (205). However, few incidents occur within the elderly cardiac population with exercise, and most of these occur in patients who have not followed their medication and diet regimens. Because exercise has an insulin-like effect, exercise itself may contribute to the incidence of hypoglycemia, particularly in patients who are also losing weight. These individuals may also exhibit lower blood pressure, which may contribute to their symptoms. But symptoms associated with what appears to be exercise-induced hypoglycemia are often also related to a combination of exercise and noncompliance to prescribed diabetic regimens.

Hypoglycemia may also result when there is an accelerated absorption of insulin from the injection site, which can occur with exercise. Accelerated absorption generally occurs when short-acting insulin is injected near the active muscles. Patients with insulin-dependent diabetes must be cautioned not to inject insulin directly into muscle groups used in exercise, because increased blood flow may increase insulin uptake and precipitate hypoglycemia. This cause of hypoglycemia is not often observed in the elderly cardiac patient population.

People with insulin-dependent diabetes have an increased risk of hypoglycemic reaction during or after exercise of high intensity and long duration (205). Hypoglycemic reactions can occur for 24 to 48 hr postexercise; thus, additional blood glucose monitoring is recommended in such cases. Additional precautions for minimizing the risk of hypoglycemic events include avoiding exercise during periods of peak insulin activity and refraining from exercising alone (205). The program staff should also inform patients about proper foot hygiene and footwear and give precautions for exercise in the heat and associated symptoms. Frequent assessment of patients using beta-blocking medications is recommended because these patients are less likely to experience hypoglycemic symptoms or angina.

Obese Patients

An exercise program for the obese elderly cardiac patient serves several functions related to overall health and fitness. Chronic exercise promotes weight management through increased caloric energy expenditure while slowing the rate of lean tissue loss that usually occurs when a person loses weight by dieting alone (205). Physical activity should also help maintain the resting metabolic rate, which assists in the rate of weight loss.

Obese subjects are usually sedentary and may have had a poor experience with exercise in the past (205). The obese patient should be interviewed to determine exercise history so that likes and dislikes related to physical activity may be discovered and appropriate goals for success determined. This process may also foster stronger relationships between staff and patients and thus may improve program adherence.

Obese patients should be able to use all exercise devices available in the standard cardiac rehabilitation exercise facility. However, some emphasis on non-weight-bearing activities initially should be considered in order to prevent muscle and joint strain and potential orthopedic injury.

Because of obesity and deconditioning, the exercise prescription for this patient group should focus on exercise duration and caloric expenditure. Exercise intensity should be less emphasized, and the exercise target heart rate should be near the low end of the standard recommended range. Increased duration and increased frequency of low-intensity activity allows for appropriate caloric expenditure over several weeks of participation and thus facilitates weight management (205). As patients adapt to physical activity, exercise intensity can be increased. But for most obese patients, exercise duration and frequency of activity continue to be most important in aiding in weight control and reducing the likelihood of physical injury.

Patients With Arthritis

Arthritis, a prevalent disease in the elderly cardiac population, can significantly limit physical activity patterns. For these patients, physical limitations associated with arthritis are often more significant than those related to the cardiovascular disorder (205). Recent literature, however, has demonstrated the potential for significant improvement in maximal oxygen uptake, muscle strength, and functional capacity following exercise training in patients with arthritis (135, 174).

Standard exercise testing methodologies can be used in elderly cardiac patients with arthritis, but because of various potential limitations, these patients are frequently unable to achieve maximal cardiovascular end points, thus reducing the sensitivity of the test in the diagnosis of CAD or changes in cardiovascular disease status. Modalities for exercise testing should focus on those joints not acutely affected by the disease.

Because many patients with arthritis have at least minimal, if not significant, limitations in physical activity associated with the disease, a staff knowledgeable about the disease process and its relationship to the prescription of exercise is essential. At the beginning, exercise should be supervised to ensure compliance and detection of arthritic flare-ups. Minor joint pain and swelling when initiating exercise is common, and ice should be routinely used on affected joints after exercise. However, actively inflamed joints indicate a high degree of disease activity and can be further aggravated with exercise (205). Exercise intensity may need to be altered frequently and progression of the exercise prescription delayed until localized aggravation subsides. In some rare instances, the exercise program may need to be completely discontinued, although some activity is desirable.

The modification and interaction of exercise intensity, frequency, duration, and progression will depend on individual disease activity and level of discomfort (205). Low-intensity activity for short periods of time requiring frequent repetition may be most appropriate for some patients. Those areas of the body not affected by the disease may be able to accomplish greater intensities of activity, which is typical of elderly rehabilitation patients in general. Patients should be encouraged to participate in some minimal amount of physical activity during periods of high disease activity, focusing on the maintenance of range of motion and avoidance of the physiological and orthopedic problems associated with inactivity.

Many patients use anti-inflammatory drugs to treat this condition, which may prevent some of the problems associated with exercise. Caution is indicated, however, because these medications may decrease the pain sensation experienced during exercise and possibly increase the risk of tissue damage (205).

There are no specific contraindications regarding modalities for exercise for these patients, although non-weight-bearing activities may receive more emphasis. Specific strengthening and flexibility exercises should be included to optimize joint stability and range of motion (205). When using stationary cycling, the patient may be able to better tolerate activity with a higher seat position, which allows for fuller extension of the knee joint, if knee joint arthritis and pain are problematic. Reduced resistance and the use of toe clips should also reduce specific stress on the knee joint as the focal point of movement.

Summary

The compilation of demographic information and patient profiles that characterize the elderly are useful in program design, development, and modification. This is particularly true because cardiac risk factors, exercise capacity, and medical presentation at entrance into exercise training are different among elderly cardiac patients than in younger patients. Also, there are wide variations in elderly cardiac patients. Although cardiac rehabilitation programs are individualized for all participants, this is an even more important consideration in designing a specific program for an elderly patient. We have less experience with the elderly cardiac population, and we need to be cognizant of the general and specific needs of these patients.

Chapter 7

Program Design Considerations

Recent advances in the care of elderly cardiac patients will probably extend longevity an additional 10 to 20 years following the initial diagnosis of CHD (119). And high-risk patients with myocardial ischemia, arrhythmias, or chronic congestive heart failure will make up a much greater percentage of participants. Health care professionals will be challenged to increase the quantity and quality of programs. Because of an increase in older patients and the differences in this population profile compared to younger patients (as was noted in chapter 6), the structure of rehabilitation programs may need to be modified.

Risk Stratification

As the number of elderly cardiac patients increases, the risk of adverse events during exercise needs to be assessed. Risk stratification for participation in an exercise program has been described for younger patients (Table 7.1) but has yet to be evaluated in the elderly cardiac patient (9, 77).

Studies presented in chapter 6 indicate that a significant number of elderly cardiac patients entering Phase II have reduced exercise capacity, exercise-induced myocardial ischemia, and complex ventricular arrhythmias. Whether these variables have similar levels of prognostic significance for the elderly in cardiac rehabilitation as for younger patients or whether other variables are more valuable remains to be determined.

Risk stratification also plays an important role in deciding between supervised and nonsupervised exercise. For the elderly, however, risk is based not only on questions of medical necessity and stability but also on nonclinical factors related

Table 7.1 Risk Stratification for Cardiac Patients

Low risk
- Uncomplicated clinical course in the hospital
- No resting or exertional evidence of myocardial ischemia
- Functional capacity of ≥6 MET
- Normal left ventricular ejection fraction (>50%)
- Absence of significant ventricular ectopy

Moderate risk
- Functional capacity of 4 to 5.9 MET
- Moderately impaired left ventricular ejection fraction (35% to 49%)

High risk
- Impaired left ventricular ejection fraction (<35%)
- Exertional hypotension
- Recurrent angina posthospitalization
- Functional capacity of <4 MET
- Exertional myocardial ischemia
- Reversible thallium defect
- Congestive heart failure during hospitalization
- Complex ventricular arrhythmias

From *Guidelines for Cardiac Rehabilitation Programs* (p. 5) by the American Association of Cardio-vascular and Pulmonary Rehabilitation, 1991, Champaign, IL: Human Kinetics. Copyright 1991 by the American Association of Cardiovascular and Pulmonary Rehabilitation. Adapted by permission.

to adherence. Elderly patients who are low risk and able to exercise independently may still need group support, some of it supervised. The interactions within a supervised group setting may be the most important factor for adherence and thus the most important factor related to successful long-term lifestyle modification.

Safety, Attendance, and Compliance

No events of morbidity or mortality during exercise have been reported among elderly cardiac patients participating in formal exercise training programs (4, 5, 278). But the data on safety may be biased because of a low-risk referral base. In addition, it is not known whether the absence of reports of untoward events suggests a low event rate or rather that not enough data on this issue is available. More experience with moderate- to high-risk elderly cardiac patients is required before we can assume that these reduced event rates are representative of the entire elderly cardiac patient population.

Attendance in elderly patients has been reported to be similar to that of younger patients, 90% versus 85%, respectively (278). The comparable or better levels of attendance may reflect the fact that the elderly may have fewer distractions, even though they may have more complicated courses resulting from CHD. Because most elderly patients are retired, it may be easier for them to participate in programs, provided that travel, class time, and economic considerations are not issues. The elderly may be enthusiastic about participation because it provides them with an enjoyable activity during the day.

Noncompliance is particularly problematic in cardiac patients because it is associated with increased risk of fatal CHD events (67). It has been estimated that 50% of patients drop out of cardiac rehabilitation programs within the first 6 months of participation (54). It has also been reported that women have more than twice the dropout rate and lower attendance than men. These observations may suggest that program staff lack knowledge about or are insensitive to the specific needs of female participants, younger or older (110, 195). In the only study reporting compliance in an elderly patient population, 6-month compliance was 40% in patients aged 75 or older (277). Of those who did not complete at least 6 months, nearly 50% discontinued for medical reasons, including cardiac and noncardiac problems. Increased compliance in this group was associated with a 5-MET or greater exercise capacity at completion of Phase II and with the ability to increase exercise training intensity during the first 3 months of training. For younger patients, predictors of noncompliance include emotional distress, low self-esteem, social introversion, blue-collar occupational status, Type A behavior, angina, and smoking behavior (44, 190). No relationship between age and compliance has been reported (170).

Increased compliance can be facilitated by choosing activities that are enjoyable and interesting (99). Programs and equipment may need to be modified for the elderly because of physical limitations. Early assessment of targeted risk factors and health-related practices is essential for successful risk modification. In addition, goal setting is especially important in programs for older cardiac patients (154). An assessment of whether patient goals are realistic is necessary; this can be determined by the patient and a cardiac rehabilitation staff member working together. Examples of areas for goal setting are presented in Table 7.2.

Economic Considerations

The impact of an aging society, the evolving economic climate, and the cost-benefit ratios of health care spanning into the next century will directly affect health care provision for the elderly. Cardiac rehabilitation programs that experience large increases in elderly patients will also be affected. The cost of supervised, telemetry-monitored, Phase II exercise programs will continue to increase, and the ability to pay will continue to be limited by out-of-pocket expenses for those on fixed incomes. Cost-effectiveness of such programs must also be related to quality of life outcomes in the elderly cardiac patient. Although little attention has been paid to these issues in this group, it is quite probable that, as with younger patients, education and physical activity will be a part of any quality of life outcome parameters. It is also likely that the elderly will not be able to afford such interventions at the current levels of cost and copayments. Rehabilitation specialists will need to develop creative methods to allow these individuals to

Table 7.2   Areas for Goal Setting Regarding Physical Activity and Health Behavior Patterns

---

Physical activity
- Formal and informal exercise programs
- Recreational activities including hobbies
- Activities of daily living
- Occupational activities

Health behavior patterns
- Smoking cessation
- Dietary patterns
  Sodium, cholesterol, saturated fats, calories, food types (fried, fatty, salty), caffeine, alcohol

Medication education
- Knowledge (type, indication, dosage)
- Adherence

Signs and symptoms
- Knowledge and understanding of angina, irregular heart beats, palpitations, dizziness

Psychosocial concerns
- Stress management
- Relaxation techniques
- Finances (personal and family)
  Health care costs
- Physical symptoms
  Sleep disturbances, headaches
- Depression
- Sexual activity
- Quality of life
- Self-esteem

Family education
- Patient's condition, family needs, family problems

Compiled from Marston (170).

participate in both lifestyle and exercise programming and, at the same time, reduce costs to both patients and programs.

One method to reduce the cost of the exercise program would be to develop and adhere to standard Phase II program exit criteria. For too long, many programs have allowed and, in some cases, encouraged participants to continue with Phase II ECG-monitored exercise sessions until their insurance reimbursement is depleted, regardless of the patient's level of activity or medical indication. Although precise criteria for an exit standard have not been identified, our experience suggests that if elderly patients can exercise at a level of 5 to 6 METs without signs or symptoms, they should be moved into the nonmonitored program and encouraged to exercise under less supervision. Advancement to Phase III can occur as early as 6 weeks after entrance into the program; some patients may advance even sooner. As mentioned previously, the elderly are at no greater risk of untoward events during exercise than are younger patients; so earlier participation in less supervised exercise programs is safe and beneficial.

The elderly must understand that they are responsible for their personal health and must be motivated to accept that responsibility. Self-motivation techniques include keeping their own exercise records, setting up and reviewing appointments for reevaluations, modifying expected outcomes based on successes and failures within the programs, and being recognized individually and within the group for achievement.

Exercise Programming

Generally, it has been our policy at the Creighton Cardiac Center not to consider age when grouping patients into exercise classes, regardless of clinical characteristics. We believe this encourages patients to interact and socialize with others of a wide range of age groups and health histories, and we hope it reduces the sense of disengagement or alienation that patients might feel at the outset of a program, especially the elderly (110). However, as the number of elderly patients continues to increase, and because data suggest that many elderly participants are limited in exercise capacity, classes for different levels of ability and clinical needs should be developed. Recently, several of our more active participants have requested to be moved into exercise classes with patients of similar physical work capacity. Because so many elderly patients are limited in ability to exercise, homogeneous grouping is an area for future consideration.

Rehabilitation professionals can do several "little things" to enable the elderly patient to participate more easily in the exercise program. Safety measures must be explained and reinforced frequently. Such measures include discussing and demonstrating appropriate procedures for treadmill exercise. Also, staff should ask elderly patients to hold onto stationary pieces of exercise equipment during upright warm-up to prevent loss of balance and falls. Frequent teaching of pulse taking and discussion of inappropriate signs or symptoms related to exertion will help the elderly gain adequate confidence in their abilities for self-monitoring. Charts and other printed directions for exercise and exercise equipment should be in large print and contain thorough explanations. These are examples of the special considerations that can enhance the exercise atmosphere for the elderly cardiac patient.

Program staff must continue to search for the most appropriate training modalities for the elderly. Adherence will be a function of patient risk and creative programming that centers around nonmonitored, less supervised, or unsupervised exercise. In some instances, walking programs may be ideal for achieving the benefits associated with physical activity, especially in this age group. The aerobic cost of walking has been documented, and although walking may not provide sufficient intensity for a training benefit in younger subjects, it can be an excellent training modality for those in their 70s, 80s, and 90s (35, 50). Walking may also decrease anxiety and depression and aid in weight control (268).

Educational Programming

Prevention of future events is an integral part of cardiac rehabilitation. Patient education, counseling, and behavior modification are important; program staff members must be trained in the skills needed to provide information regarding health-related behaviors, in measurement of outcomes of these behavioral interventions, and in periodic reinforcement for the elderly (37).

Patient education and lifestyle modification are influenced by the characteristics of the patient population. In chapter 6, it was demonstrated that the elderly possess specific needs related to both physical activity and lifestyle modification. Program staff need to consider these needs in modifying educational programs for the elderly. For example, dietary and nutritional interventional programs may need to be reviewed and revised because many patients are elderly, overweight, and hypertensive.

Elderly cardiac patients also have other limitations that must be considered. For example, patients with sight or hearing limitations may have specific needs based on their ability to process information. Some may prefer a traditional seminar or lecture presentation to obtain information, whereas others may prefer multimedia approaches including videotapes and written materials that can be reviewed in a formal group setting or at home. Still others may enjoy workshops that involve a hands-on approach, especially on dietary topics such as weight loss and limiting fat and sodium intake. This type of presentation may be particularly suited to demonstrations of food preparation and stress reduction. Combinations of these techniques should be most effective (268).

Quality of Life

Quality of life is an important aspect of program outcomes. This fact is especially significant for the elderly cardiac patient. Whereas exercise and health-related education programs for younger patients have resulted in decreased mortality levels, a reduction in mortality levels may be less important for the elderly than more basic issues (191). These include a sense of well-being, life satisfaction, and the ability to participate in valued activities in the home, the workplace, or the community (110, 268).

Evaluating the quality of life can be highly subjective. The values and expectations of the participants will affect program outcomes and must be defined. The expected outcomes—which may be related to recovery and survival—and the desired levels of health, independence, and productivity are major factors in maintaining an effective and individualized rehabilitation program (268). Determining desired patient outcomes is the first step in designing the program.

The cardiac rehabilitation program may provide additional outlets for enhancing the patient's life satisfaction. Most elderly cardiac participants are retired, so some patients use the rehabilitation program for reasons other than exercise and education. The elderly may belong to a program to fill the gaps in daily routine, or they may view exercise and education classes as significant social opportunities. Consequently, many patients can be active in the program beyond the role of patient. They can be asked to assume responsibilities such as organizing patient education meetings or social events that center around the rehabilitation program, developing support groups, serving on the program's board of directors, or assisting with orientations. Along with their spouses, patients can be of immeasurable value, involving themselves in healthful activities in the community as well as within the rehabilitation program itself.

Summary

The time has long passed for excluding candidates from outpatient cardiac rehabilitation on the basis of age. As the number of elderly patients increases, cardiac rehabilitation professionals are challenged to provide meaningful and valuable programs and to determine ways of making these programs available. Independence is an important concern for the elderly, those who care for them, and those who may be responsible for the costs of health, sickness, and dependence. We must continue to evaluate the specific needs of this group and respond wherever possible with new and innovative approaches to enhance recruitment and maintain adherence to programs of physical activity and lifestyle management.

Warm-Up, Stretching, and Flexibility Exercises

It is important to correctly perform the warm-up, moving slowly and breathing properly through each exercise. This prepares the cardiovascular and muscular systems for the exercise session and enhances flexibility. Patients should hold each stretch for 10 to 12 seconds and repeat exercises on the opposite side where applicable. But because the elderly patients' bodies may be quite inflexible when they begin the program, they do not need to conform exactly to the body positions illustrated in the following examples. As with all other aspects of the exercise program, an individualized approach is appropriate. Also, patients may tend to hold their breath or strain during these activities, and the rehabilitation staff should guard against these tendencies.

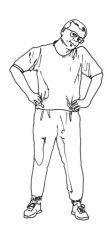

Neck

The patient moves the head side to side laterally 5 to 10 times. This exercise may be modified by turning the head as if attempting to look behind and holding at the point where the head cannot be turned any farther.

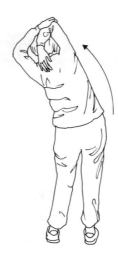

Shoulders and back

The patient raises one arm and drops the hand behind the head. Grasping the elbow with the opposite hand, the patient bends gently to the side opposite the raised elbow.

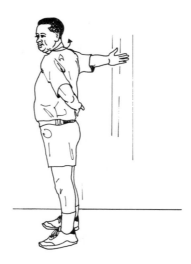

Shoulders

Standing with one side next to a wall, the patient places the near palm on the wall with arm outstretched, turning the head away from the outstretched arm. The arm opposite the wall should be tucked behind the back.

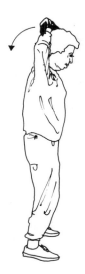

Shoulders

The patient grasps a towel overhead with arms outstretched, slowly lowering arms behind the head and then the shoulders, increasing the bend in the elbows. The stretch should be held at the point where the arms can no longer move down comfortably.

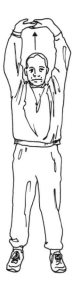

Shoulders and arms

With fingers interlocked overhead, the patient stretches the arms up.

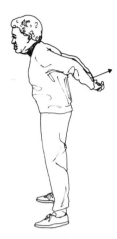

Shoulders and arms

The patient clasps hands behind the buttocks and attempts to raise arms up and away from the body without bending forward at the waist.

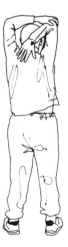

Shoulders and triceps

The patient raises one arm and drops the hand behind the head. Grasping the elbow with the opposite hand, the patient pushes the raised elbow toward the opposite shoulder.

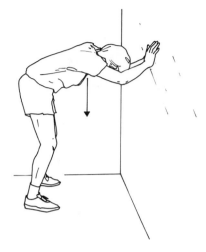

Back

The patient stands about 18 inches from a wall, facing it, with knees slightly bent and places hands against the wall slightly above waist level. The patient bends at the waist and pushes the face and chest toward the floor. The stretch should be held at the point where shoulders are below the hands.

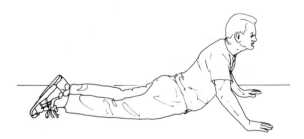

Shoulders and trunk

Lying front-down on the floor, the patient places the hands underneath the shoulders. The patient then pushes the torso up from the hands until elbows are fully extended, keeping pelvis and hips on the floor.

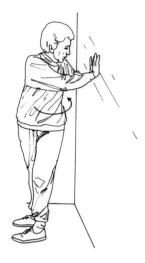

Trunk

The patient stands with back 8 to 12 inches from a wall. The patient gently twists toward the wall and places hands there, then continues to twist in the same direction.

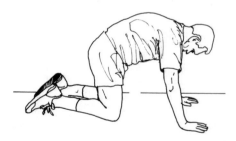

Trunk

From a position on hands and knees on the floor, the patient arches the back, attempting to touch chin to chest.

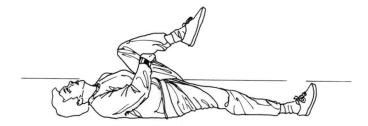

Back

Lying on the back on the floor, the patient grasps behind the thigh with both hands and pulls the knee toward the chin.

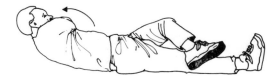

Trunk

Lying on the back on the floor with arms at sides, the patient crosses one ankle over the opposite knee. The patient crosses the arm opposite the bent knee over the chest, allowing the shoulder to come off the ground and gently rotating the torso in that direction.

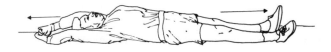

Back

Lying on the back on the floor with arms raised overhead, the patient stretches to lengthen the body as far as possible.

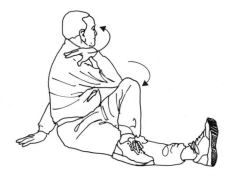

Trunk and buttocks

Sitting on the floor with legs extended straight forward, the patient crosses one leg over the opposite knee, resting on the arm on the bent-leg side for support. The patient twists body and head gently in the direction of the support arm. The patient stretches by pressing the free elbow against the outside of the bent knee.

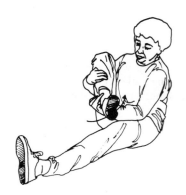

Buttocks

Sitting with the legs extended straight ahead, the patient bends one knee, grasps the ankle, and pulls the foot toward the chest.

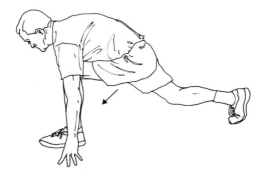

Hips

The patient crouches on the ground as if waiting to start a race (front leg bent, rear leg extended behind the body, both hands on the floor for support). The patient gradually shifts weight to the front leg, pushing the hips forward and toward the ground.

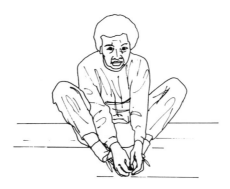

Inner thighs

Sitting on the ground, the patient bends the knees and places the soles of the feet together. The patient then attempts to push the knees toward the ground without using the elbows.

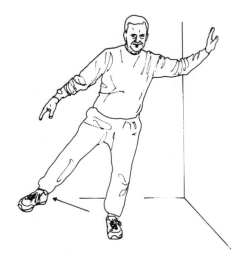

Hips

Standing with one side about 2 feet from a wall, the patient places the near hand against the wall for balance and lifts the far leg to the side.

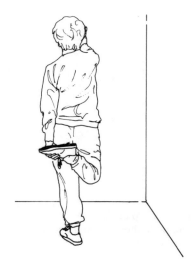

Front thigh

The patient stands about 18 inches from a wall, facing it, and places one hand against it for support. The patient reaches the other hand behind to grasp the opposite foot and pulls the foot up.

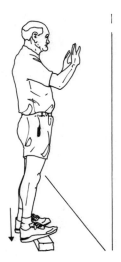

Lower leg

The patient stands on a block or raised surface about 18 inches from a wall. Using the wall for support and balance, the patient lowers the heels toward the floor.

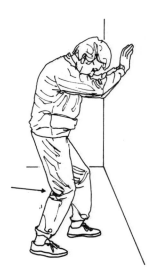

Lower leg

The patient stands facing a wall with legs staggered (front leg 12 to 14 inches from the wall). With hands on the wall for support, the patient attempts to push the back knee toward the wall, keeping both heels on the ground.

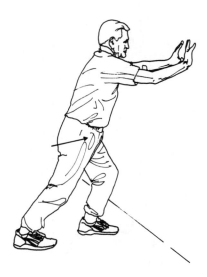

Lower leg

The patient stands facing a wall with legs staggered (front leg 12 to 14 inches from the wall, back leg straight) and with hands on the wall for support. The patient attempts to push the hips toward the wall.

Home Exercise Program Log Book

Name _____ Date _____

Introduction

This program was designed to guide your physical activity at home. The exercise prescription was written especially for you. Please read carefully and record your progress. Call regarding questions or concerns.

Benefits of Exercise

1. Reduced symptoms associated with exercise
2. More efficient use of oxygen
3. Lowered resting and exercise heart rate
4. Lowered resting and exercise blood pressure
5. Assistance with weight loss
6. Improved levels of various blood fats
7. Improved exercise capacity
8. Improved general sense of well-being

General Exercise Precautions

- Your pulse rate is your most important exercise guideline. Know your target heart rate and how to take your pulse.
- Do not exercise if resting heart rate exceeds target heart rate (THR) or resting heart rate is greater than 100 beats per min.
- Do not exercise during illness or fever.
- Do not exercise outdoors if temperature is above 95 °F or wind chill is below 0 °F. Use caution if temperature is above 85 °F or wind chill is below

20 °F. Consider indoor alternatives such as shopping malls for walking, or substitute stationary cycling at home.

- Exercise before eating, or allow 1 to 2 hrs after eating.
- Avoid caffeine, alcohol, and smoking.
- Postpone exercise at times when you are emotionally upset or excessively fatigued.
- Exercise should be rhythmical and constant; stop only to check your pulse or if symptoms occur.
- Do not exercise in isolated areas alone. Exercise is more fun with a buddy!

Warm-Up and Cool-Down Exercises

Each cardiac rehabilitation session starts with warm-up exercises. It is important to correctly perform the warm-up, moving slowly and breathing properly through each exercise. The entire warm-up lasts 5 to 10 minutes and prepares the cardiovascular and muscular systems for the exercise session. The following exercises provide a good warm-up:

1. Neck circles—Slowly move the head side to side in a half-circle; 5 to 10 times.
2. Shoulder shrugs—Raise and lower shoulders; 5 to 10 times.
3. Chest stretch—Cross the arms in front of the body, parallel to the floor, and then pull the arms back, 5 to 10 times.
4. Arm circles—Working one arm at a time, move arm through the complete range of motion, and then reverse; 5 times each direction.
5. Side-to-side stretches—Bend side to side in lateral plane; 5 to 10 times.
6. Trunk circles—Rotate the trunk in one direction, and then reverse; 5 times each direction.
7. Side lunges—Step to the side and slightly bend one knee, not allowing it to pass beyond the toe; 5 times each side.
8. Knee bends—Slightly bend knees, holding a support as needed; 5 to 10 times.
9. Heel raises—From standing position, shift weight up on toes; 5 to 10 times.
10. Heel-toe rock—Shift weight from heels to toes, holding a support as needed; 5 to 10 times.

Slow down or decrease exercise intensity when you have these symptoms:

1. Unusual fatigue
2. Shortness of breath
3. Beginning symptoms of angina
4. Any unusual joint or muscle pain or cramping

Stop exercising when you have these symptoms:

1. Increasing pain, pressure, tightness or fullness in the chest, jaw, neck, upper shoulders, or arms*

2. Light-headedness or dizziness
3. Extreme shortness of breath
4. Extreme weakness or fatigue
5. Cold sweat
6. Palpitations, fluttering, or irregular heart beat
7. Nausea or vomiting

*If symptoms of angina do not stop with the cessation of exercise, place a nitroglycerin (NTG) tablet under the tongue. Wait 5 min; if there is no relief, repeat. If there is still no relief, take a third NTG. If you still have no relief after 3 NTG, call or have someone drive you to the nearest hospital emergency room. If you have questions about your exercise program or symptoms, please call

_____ .

Exercise Prescription

Mode (type of exercise) _____

_____

_____

_____

Intensity (how hard to exercise)

Warm-up heart rate: _____

_____

Training or target heart rate: _____

_____

Cool-down heart rate: _____

_____

The highest your heart rate should be at any time is _____

_____

Duration (how long to exercise)

Warm-up (minutes): _____

Exercise training (minutes): _____

Cool-down (minutes): _____

Frequency (how often to exercise) _____

_____

_____

Progression: See Progression of Exercise at the end of this booklet if needed.

Record specific information regarding each daily exercise session in the Daily Log at the end of this booklet.

Remember, this program has been designed specifically for you as of _____ . It will need periodic review and revision, especially if there are any changes in your medications or condition.

Your program should be re-evaluated at the following times:

- Every 6 months
- After any type of exercise stress test
- When there are changes in your medications, especially heart drugs
- When you have changes or new onset of chest pain

_____

_____

_____

_____

Program staff   Phone extension

_____

_____

Daily Log

Training heart rate _____

Date	Mode	Resting pulse	Maximum pulse	Total time	Comments/ symptoms

Progression of Exercise

	Warm-up (min)	Exercise training (min)	Cool-down (min)
Week ___			
Week ___			
Week ___			
Week ___			
Week ___			
Week ___			
Week ___			
Week ___			

Appendix B adapted from the *Outpatient Cardiac Rehabilitation Program Home Exercise Booklet* by Teresa Lynch and Mark Williams at Omaha, NE: Creighton University School of Medicine, Division of Cardiology, Cardiovascular Disease Prevention and Rehabilitation Program.

References

1. Abrams, W.B. Cardiovascular drugs in the elderly. Chest. 98:980-986; 1990.
2. Ackerman, R.F.; Dry, T.J.; Edwards, J.E. Relationship with various factors to the degree of coronary atherosclerosis in women. Circulation. 1:1345-1354; 1950.
3. Adams, G.M.; deVries, H.A. Physiological effects of an exercise training regimen upon women aged 42 to 79. Journal of Gerontology. 28:50-55; 1973.
4. Ades, P.A.; Grunvald, M.H. Cardiopulmonary exercise testing before and after conditioning in older coronary patients. American Heart Journal. 120:585-589; 1990.
5. Ades, P.A.; Hanson, J.S.; Gunther, J.G.S.; Tonino, R.P. Exercise conditioning in the elderly coronary patient. Journal of the American Geriatric Society. 35:121-124; 1987.
6. Ades, P.A.; Waldman, M.L.; McCann, W.J.; Weaver, S.O. Predictors of cardiac rehabilitation participation in older patients. Archives of Internal Medicine. 152:1022-1035; 1992.
7. Ades, P.A.; Waldman, M.L., Pol, D.A.; Coflesky, J.T. Referral patterns and exercise response in the rehabilitation of female coronary patients aged 62 years. American Journal of Cardiology. 69:1422-1425; 1992.
8. Aloia, J.F.; Cohn, S.H.; Ostuni, J.D.; Cane, R.; Ellis, K. Prevention of involutional bone loss by exercise. Annals of Internal Medicine. 89:356-358; 1978.
9. American Association of Cardiovascular and Pulmonary Rehabilitation. Guidelines for cardiac rehabilitation programs. Champaign, IL: Human Kinetics Books; 1991:1-8.
10. American College of Cardiology/American Heart Association Task Force on Assessment of Cardiovascular Procedures (Subcommittee on Exercise Testing). Guidelines for exercise testing. Journal of the American College of Cardiology. 8:725-738; 1986.
11. American Heart Association. An active partnership for the health of your heart. Dallas: American Heart Association; 1990.
12. Aniansson, A.; Gustafsson, E. Physical training in elderly men with special reference to quadriceps, muscle, strength, and morphology. Clinical Physiology. 1:87-98; 1981.
13. Aronow, W.S.; Ahn, C.; Kronzon, I.; Koenigsberg, M. Congestive heart failure, coronary events and atherothrombotic brain infarction in elderly blacks and whites with systemic hypertension and with and without echocardiographic and electrocardiographic evidence of left ventricular hypertrophy. American Journal of Cardiology. 67:295-299; 1991.

14. Aronow, W.S.; Herzig, A.H.; Etienne, F.; D'Alba, P.; Ronquillo, J. 41-month follow-up of risk factors correlated with new coronary events in 708 elderly patients. Journal of the American Geriatric Society. 37:501-506; 1989.

15. Aronow, W.S.; Kronzon, I. Prevalence of coronary risk factors in elderly blacks and whites. Journal of the American Geriatric Society. 39:567-570; 1991.

16. Aronow, W.S.; Sales, F.F.; Etienne, F.; Lee, N.H. Prevalence of peripheral arterial disease and its correlation with risk factors for peripheral arterial disease in elderly patients in a long-term health care facility. American Journal of Cardiology. 62:644-646; 1988.

17. Aronow, W.S.; Starling, L.; Etienne, F.; D'Alba, P.; Edwards, M.; Lee, N.H.; Parungao, R.F. Risk factors for coronary artery disease in persons older than 62 years in a long-term health care facility. American Journal of Cardiology. 57:518-520; 1986.

18. Arvan, S. Exercise performance of the high risk, acute myocardial infarction patient after cardiac rehabilitation. American Journal of Cardiology. 62:197-201; 1988.

19. Asmussen, E. Similarities and dissimilarities between static and dynamic exercise. Circulation Research. [Suppl. 1] 48:3-10; 1981.

20. Åstrand, I.; Åstrand, P.O. Aerobic work performance: a review. In. Folinsbee, L.B. ed. Environmental stress: individual human adaptations. New York: Academic Press; 1978:149-163.

21. Åstrand, P.O. Quantification of exercise capability and evaluation of physical capacity in men. Progress in Cardiovascular Diseases. 19:51-67; 1976.

22. Avolio, A.P.; Deng, F.Q.; Li, W.Q.; Luo, Y.F.; Huang, Z.D.; Xing, L.F.; O'Rourke, M.F. Effects of aging on arterial distensibility in populations with high and low prevalence of hypertension: comparison between urban and rural communities. Circulation. 71:202-210; 1985.

23. Badger, J.M.; Morris, P.L. Observations of a support group for automatic implantable cardioverter-defibrillator recipients and their spouses. Heart and Lung. 18:238-243; 1989.

24. Baechle, T.; Williams, M.; Petratis, M.; Ryschon, K.; Worth, J.; Angelillo, V. Cardiovascular response to arm, leg, and combined arm and leg exercise in males and females. Medicine and Science In Sports and Exercise. [Abstract]. 15:109; 1983.

25. Baechle, T.R.; Groves, B.R. Weight training: steps to success. Champaign, IL: Leisure Press; 1992:141-151.

26. Balady, G.J.; Weiner, D.A. Exercise testing in healthy elderly subjects and elderly patients with cardiac disease. Journal of Cardiopulmonary Rehabilitation. 9:35-39; 1989.

27. Barclay, L.L.; Weiss, E.M.; Mattis, S.; Bond, O.; Blass, J.P. Unrecognized cognitive impairment in cardiac rehabilitation patients. Journal of the American Geriatric Society. 36:22-28; 1988.

28. Barnard, R.J.; MacAlpin, R.; Kattus, A.A.; Buckberg, G.D. Ischemic response to sudden strenuous exercise in healthy men. Circulation. 48:936-942; 1973.

29. Barrett-Connor, E.; Suarez, L.; Khaw, K.T.; Criqui, M.H.; Wingard, D.L. Ischemic heart disease risk factors after age 50. Journal of Chronic Diseases. 37:903-908; 1984.

30. Barry, A.; Steinmetz, J.; Page, H.; Rodahl, K. The effects of physical conditioning on older individuals: II. Motor performance and cognitive function. Journal of Gerontology. 21:192-199; 1966.

31. Bayer, A.J.; Chadha, J.S.; Farag, R.R.; Pathy, M.S.J. Changing presentation of myocardial infarction with increasing old age. Journal of the American Geriatric Society. 34:263-266; 1986.

32. Beller, G.A. Pharmacologic stress testing. Journal of the American Medical Association. 265:633-638; 1991.

33. Ben-Ari, E.; Kellerman, J.J. Physiologic and perceptual responses to low and moderate training intensities in two different groups of coronary patients. Journal of Cardiac Rehabilitation. 2:127-132; 1982.

34. Benestad, A.M. Trainability of old men. Acta Medica Scandinavia. 178:321-327; 1965.

35. Blair, S.N.; Kohl, H.W.; Paffenbarger, D.R., Jr.; Clark, D.G.; Cooper, K.H.; Bibbons, L.W. Physical fitness and all-cause mortality: a prospective study of healthy men and women. Journal of the American Medical Association. 262:2395-2401; 1989.

36. Blumenthal, J.A. Psychologic assessment in cardiac rehabilitation. Journal of Cardiopulmonary Rehabilitation. 5:208-215; 1985.

37. Blumenthal, J.A.; Califf, R.; Williams, S.; Hindman, M. Cardiac rehabilitation: a new frontier for behavioral medicine. Journal of Cardiac Rehabilitation. 3:637-656; 1983.

38. Blumenthal, J.A.; Emery, C.F.; Madden, D.J.; Coleman, R.E.; Riddle, M.W.; Schniebolk, S.; Cobb, F.R.; Sullivan, M.J.; Higginbotham, M.B. Effects of exercise training on cardiorespiratory function in men and women > 60 years of age. American Journal of Cardiology. 67:633-639; 1991.

39. Blumenthal, J.A.; Emery, C.F.; Madden, D.J.; George, L.K.; Coleman, R.E.; Riddle, M.W.; McKee, D.C.; Williams, R.S. Cardiovascular and behavioral effects or aerobic exercise training in healthy older men and women. Journal of Gerontology. [Suppl. M] 44:147-157; 1989.

40. Blumenthal, J.A.; Emery, C.F.; Rejeski, W.J. The effects of exercise training on psychosocial functioning after myocardial infarction. Journal of Cardiopulmonary Rehabilitation. 8:183-193; 1988.

41. Blumenthal, J.A.; Madden, D.J. The effects of aerobic exercise training, age, and physical fitness on memory-search performance. Psychology and Aging. 3:280-285; 1988.

42. Blumenthal, J.A.; Schocker, D.D.; Needels, T.L.; Hindle, P. Psychological and physiological effects of physical conditioning on the elderly. Journal of Psychomotor Research. 26:505-510; 1982.

43. Blumenthal, J.A.; Williams, R.S.; Needels, T.; Wallace, A. Psychological changes accompany aerobic exercise in healthy middle-aged adults. Psycho-motor Medicine. 44:529-536; 1982.

44. Blumenthal, J.A.; Williams, R.S.; Wallace, A.G.; Williams, R.B.; Needels, T.L. Physiological and psychological variables predict compliance to pre-scribed exercise therapy in patients recovering from myocardial infarction. Psychomotor Medicine. 44:519-527; 1982.

45. Botwinick, J. Intellectual abilities. In: Birren, J.E.; Schaie, K.W., eds. Hand-book of the psychology of aging. New York: Van Nostrand Reinhold; 1977:580-605.

46. Botwinick, J.E.; Thompson, L.W. Age differences in reaction time: an artifact? Gerontologist. 8:25-28; 1978.

47. Boyer, J.L.; Kasch, F.W. Exercise therapy in hypertension. Journal of the American Medical Association. 211:1168-1171; 1970.

48. Brandfonbrener, M.; Landowne, M.; Shock, N.W. Changes in cardiac output with age. Circulation. 12:557-566; 1955.

49. Bruce, R.A.; Fisher, L.D.; Cooper, N.M.; Gey, G.O. Separation of effects of cardiovascular disease and age on ventricular function with maximal exercise. American Journal of Cardiology. 34:757-763; 1974.

50. Bruce, R.A.; Larson, E.B.; Stratton, J. Physical fitness, functional aerobic capacity, and responses to physical training or bypass surgery in coronary patients. Journal of Cardiopulmonary Rehabilitation. 9:24-34; 1989.

51. Butler, R.M.; Beierwaltes, W.H.; Rodgers, F.J. The cardiovascular response to circuit weight training in patients with coronary diseases. Journal of Cardiopulmonary Rehabilitation. 7:402-409; 1987.

52. Butler, R.N.; Lewis, M. Aging and mental health. St. Louis: C.V. Mosby; 1977.

53. Carlson, L.A.; Rosenhamer, G. Reduction of mortality in the Stockholm Ischemic Heart Disease Secondary Prevention Study by combined treatment with clofibrate and nicotinic acid. Acta Medica Scandinavia. 223:405-418; 1988.

54. Carmody, T.; Senner, J.; Matinow, M.; Matarazzo, J. Physical exercise rehabilitation: long-term drop-out rate in cardiac patients. Journal of Behav-ioral Medicine. 3:113-168; 1980.

55. Castelli, W.P.; Wilson, P.W.F.; Levy, D.; Anderson, K. Cardiovascular risk factors in the elderly. American Journal of Cardiology. 63:12H-19H; 1989.

56. Cerebral Embolism Task Force. Cardiogenic brain embolism. Archives of Neurology. 43:71-84; 1986.

57. Checkett, J.H. Outpatient program: community based. In: Fardy, P.S.; Ben-nett, J.L.; Reitz, N.L.; Williams, M.A., eds. Cardiac rehabilitation: implica-tions for the nurse and other health professionals. St. Louis: Mosby; 1980:248-262.

58. Chung, E.K. Exercise electrocardiography practical approach. 2nd ed. Balti-more: Williams & Wilkins; 1983.

59. Cole, J.P.; Ellestad, M.H. Significance of chest pain during treadmill exercise: correlation with coronary events. American Journal of Cardiology. 41:227-232; 1978.

60. Connolly, D.C.; Elveback, L.R.; Oxman, H.A. Coronary heart disease in residents of Rochester, Minnesota, 1950-1975: III. Effect of hypertension and its treatment on survival of patients with coronary artery disease. Mayo Clinic Proceedings. 58:249-254; 1983.

61. Cononie, C.C.; Graves, J.E.; Pollock, M.L.; Phillips, M.I.; Sumners, C.; Hagberg, J.M. Effect of exercise training on blood pressure in 70- to 79-yr-old men and women. Medicine and Science in Sports and Exercise. 23:505-511; 1991.

62. The CONSENSUS Trial Study Group. Effects of enalapril on mortality in severe congestive heart failure: results of the Cooperative North Scandinavian Enalapril Survival Study. New England Journal of Medicine. 316:1429-1435; 1987.

63. Conway, J.; Wheeler, R.; Hammerstedt, R. Sympathetic nervous activity during exercise in relation to age. Cardiovascular Research. 5:577-581; 1977.

64. Cooper, D.K.; Valladares, B.K.; Futterman, L.G. Care of the patient with the automatic implantable cardioverter defibrillator: a guide for nurses. Heart and Lung. 16:640-648; 1987.

65. The Coronary Drug Project Research Group. Cigarette smoking as a risk factor in men with a prior history of myocardial infarction. Journal of Chronic Diseases. 32:415-425; 1979.

66. The Coronary Drug Project Research Group. Blood pressure in survivors of myocardial infarction. Journal of the American College of Cardiology. 4:1135-1147; 1984.

67. The Coronary Drug Project Research Group. Influence of adherence to treatment and response of cholesterol on mortality in the Coronary Drug Project. New England Journal of Medicine. 303:1038-1041; 1980.

68. Council On Scientific Affairs, American Heart Association. Exercise programs for the elderly. Journal of the American Medical Association. 252:544-546; 1984.

69. Craik, F.I.M. Age differences in human memory. In: Birren, J.E.; Schaie, K.W., eds. Handbook of the psychology of aging. New York: Van Nostrand Reinhold; 1977:384-420.

70. Cunningham, D.A.; Rechnitzer, P.A.; Howard, J.H.; Donner, A.P. Exercise training of men at retirement: a clinical trial. Journal of Gerontology. 42:17-23; 1987.

71. Das, D.N.; Fleg, J.L.; Lakatta, E.G. The effect of age on the components of atrioventricular conduction in normal man. American Journal of Cardiology. [Abstract]. [Suppl. 2] 49:1031; 1982.

72. Davey, C.P. Physical exertion and mental performance. Ergonomics. 16:595-599; 1973.

73. Davis, J.A.; Frank, M.H.; Whipp, B.J.; Wasserman, K. Anaerobic threshold alterations caused by endurance training in middle-aged men. Journal of Applied Physiology. 46:1039-1046; 1979.

74. Dayton, S.; Pearce, M.L.; Hashimoto, S.; Dixon, W.J.; Tomiyasu, U. A controlled clinical trial of a diet high in unsaturated fat in preventing complications of atherosclerosis. Circulation. 40:II1-II63; 1969.

75. Deanfield, J.E.; Maseri, A.; Selwyn, A.P.; Ribeiro, P.; Chierchia, S.; Kirkler, S.; Morgan, M. Myocardial ischemia during daily life in patients with stable angina: its relation to symptoms and heart rate changes. Lancet. 2:753-758; 1983.

76. DeBusk, R.F.; Baldez, R.; Houston, N.; Haskell, W. Cardiovascular responses to dynamic and static efforts soon after myocardial infarction: application to occupational work assessment. Circulation. 58:368-375; 1978.

77. DeBusk, R.F.; Haskell, W.L.; Miller, N.H.; Berra, K.; Taylor, C.B.; Berger, W.E.; Lew, H. Medically directed at-home rehabilitation soon after clinically uncomplicated acute myocardial infarction: a new model for patient care. American Journal of Cardiology. 55:251-257; 1985.

78. Deckers, J.W.; Fioretti, P.; Brower, R.W.; Simoons, M.L.; Baardaman, T.; Hugenholtz, P.G. Ineligibility for pre-discharge exercise testing after myocardial infarction in the elderly: implications for prognosis. European Heart Journal. [Suppl. E]. 5:97-100; 1984.

79. Deckers, J.W.; Simoons, M.L.; Fioretti, P. The value of exercise testing in elderly patients. Geriatric Cardiovascular Medicine. 1:89-93; 1988.

80. Dehn, M.M.; Bruce, A. Longitudinal variations in maximal oxygen uptake with age and activity. Journal of Applied Physiology. 33:805-807; 1972.

81. Detry, J.M.R.; Bruce, R.A. Divergent effects of physical training and nitro-glycerine in coronary heart disease. Annals of Internal Medicine. 78:819-825; 1971.

82. deVries, H.A. Physiological effects of an exercise training regimen upon men aged 52 to 88. Journal of Gerontology. 25:325-336; 1970.

83. deVries, H.A. Physiology of exercise for physical education and athletics. 2nd ed. Dubuque, IA: William C. Brown; 1986.

84. deVries, H.A.; Adams, G.M. Comparison of exercise responses in old and young men. Journal of Gerontology. 27:344-348; 1972.

85. Doan, A.E.; Peterson, D.R.; Blackman, J.R.; Bruce, R.A. Myocardial ischemia after maximal exercise in health men. American Heart Journal. 69:11-21; 1965.

86. Dustman, R.E.; Ruhling, R.O.; Russell, E.M.; Shearer, D.E.; Bonekat, W.; Shigeoka, J.W.; Wood, J.S.; Bradfort, D.C. Aerobic exercise training and improved neuropsychological function of older individuals. Neurobiology and Aging. 5:35-42; 1984.

87. Ehsani, A.A. Cardiovascular adaptations to exercise training in the elderly. Federal Proceedings. 46:1840-1843; 1987.

88. Ekblom, B. Effective physical training on oxygen transport system in man. Acta Physiologica Scandinavia. [Suppl. 328]. 77:9-45; 1969.

89. Ekblom, B.; Astrand, P.O.; Saltin, B.; Stenberg, J.; Wallstrom, B. Effective training on circulatory response to exercise. Journal of Applied Physiology. 24:518-528; 1968.

90. Elia, E.A. Exercise and the elderly. Clinics In Sports Medicine. 10:141-155; 1991.

91. Ellestad, M.H. Stress testing principles and practice. 3rd ed. Philadelphia: F.A. Davis; 1986.

92. Elsayed, M.; Ismail, A.H.; Young, R.J. Intellectual differences of adult men related to age and physical fitness before and after an exercise program. Journal of Gerontology. 35:383-387; 1980.

93. Elveback, L.; Lie, J.T. Continued high prevalence of coronary artery disease at autopsy in Olmstead County, Minnesota, 1950-1970. Circulation. 70:345-349; 1984.

94. Emery, C.F.; Pinder, S.L.; Blumenthal, J.A. Psychological effects of exercise among elderly cardiac patients. Journal of Cardiopulmonary Rehabilitation. 9:46-53; 1989.

95. Fardy, P.S.; Doll, N.E.; Taylor, J.W. Effects of two years exercise training in patients with diagnosed coronary artery disease. Medicine and Science in Sports and Exercise. [Abstract]. 12:100; 1980.

96. Ferguson, R.J.; Cote, P.; Bourassa, M.G.; Corbara, F. Coronary blood flow during isometric and dynamic exercise in angina pectoris patients. Journal of Cardiac Rehabilitation. 1:21-27; 1981.

97. Fiatarone, M.A.; Marks, E.C.; Ryan, N.D.; Meredith, C.N.; Lipsitz, L.A.; Evans, W.J. High intensity strength training in nonagenarians: effects on skeletal muscle. Journal of the American Medical Association. 263:3029-3034; 1990.

98. Fioretti, P.; Deckers, J.W.; Brower, R.W.; Simoons, M.L.; Beelen, J.A.J.M.; Hugenholtz, P.G. Pre-discharge stress test after myocardial infarction in the old age: results and prognostic value. European Heart Journal. [Suppl. E]. 5:101-104; 1984.

99. Fitzgerald, P.L. Exercise for the elderly. Medical Clinics of North America. 69:189-196; 1985.

100. Fleg, J.L.; Gerstenblith, G.; Lakatta, E.G. Pathophysiology of the aging heart and circulation. In: F.H. Messeril, ed. Cardiovascular disease in the elderly. Boston: Martinus Nijhoff Publishing; 1988:9-36.

101. Fleg, J.L.; Kennedy, H.L. Cardiac arrthymias in a healthy elderly population: detection by 24-hour ambulatory electrocardiography. Chest. 81:302-307; 1982.

102. Folkins, C.H.; Lynch, S.; Gardner, M.M. Psychological fitness as a function of physical fitness. Archives of Physical Medicine and Rehabilitation. 53:503-508; 1972.

103. Folkins, C.H.; Sime, W.F. Physical fitness training in mental health. American Psychologist. 36:371-389; 1981.

104. Fordyce, W.; McMahon, R.; Rainwater, G.; Jackins, S.; Questad, K.; Murphy, T.; De Lateur, B. Pain complaint: exercise performance relationship in chronic pain. Pain. 10:311-321; 1981.

105. Froelicher, V.; Perdue, S.; Pewen, W.; Risch, M. Application of meta-analysis using an electronic spread sheet to exercise testing in patients after myocardial infarction. American Journal of Medicine. 83:1045-1054; 1987.

106. Froelicher, V.F. Exercise testing and training. 2nd ed. Chicago: Mosby Yearbook Medical Publishers; 1987.

107. Frontera, W.R.; Meredith, C.N.; O'Reilly, K.P.; Knuttgen, H.G.; Evans, W.J. Strength conditioning in older men: skeletal muscle hypertrophy and improved function. Journal of Applied Physiology. 64:1038-1044; 1988.

108. Fung, A.Y.; Gallagher, K.P.; Buda, A.J. The physiologic basis of dobutamine as compared with dipyridamole stress interventions in the assessment of critical coronary stenosis. Circulation. 76:943-951; 1987.

109. Gardin, J.M.; Henry, W.L.; Savage, D.D.; Ware, J.H.; Burns, C.; Borer, J.S. Echocardiographic measurements in normal subjects: evaluation of an adult population without clinically apparent heart disease. Journal of Clinical Ultrasound. 7:349-447; 1979.

110. Gentry, W.D.; Crews, W.D., Jr.; Brooks, S.J. Psychosocial aspects of rehabilitation of elderly coronary patients. Geriatric Cardiovascular Medicine. 1:111-114; 1988.

111. Gerson, M.C.; Moore, E.N.; Ellis, K. Systemic affects and safety of intravenous dipyridamole in elderly patients with suspected coronary artery disease. American Journal of Cardiology. 60:1399-1401; 1987.

112. Gerstenblith, G.; Frederiksen, J.; Yin, F.C.P. Echocardiography assessment of a normal adult aging population. Circulation. 56:273-278; 1977.

113. Ghilarducci, L.E.; Holly, R.G.; Amsterdam, E.A. Effects of high resistance training in coronary artery disease. American Journal of Cardiology. 64:866-870; 1989.

114. Glover, D.R.; Robinson, C.S.; Murray, R.G. Diagnostic exercise testing in 104 patients over 65 years of age. European Heart Journal. [Suppl. E]. 5:59-62; 1984.

115. Gottlieb, S.O.; Gerstenblith, G. Silent myocardial ischemia in the elderly: current concepts. Geriatrics. 43:29-34; 1988.

116. Granath, A.; Jonsson, B.; Strandell, T. Circulation in healthy old men studied by right heart catheterization at rest and during exercise in a supine and sitting position. Acta Medica Scandinavia. 176:425-446; 1964.

117. Griest, J.H.; Klein, M.; Eischens, R.R.; Faris, J.W.; Gurman, S.S.; Morgan, W.P. Running as a treatment for depression. Comparative Psychiatry. 20:41-54; 1979.

118. Gupta, N.C.; Esterbrooks, D.; Mohiuddin, S.; Hilleman, D.; Sunderland, J.; Shiue, C.Y.; Frick, M.P. Adenosine in myocardial perfusion imaging using positron emission tomography. American Heart Journal. 122:293-301; 1991.

119. Guralnik, J.M.; FitzSimmons, S.C. Aging in America: a demographic perspective. Cardiology Clinics. 4:175-183; 1986.
120. Gutin, B. The effect of increase in physical fitness on mental ability following physical and mental stress. Research Quarterly. 37:211-220; 1966.
121. Hagberg, J.M. Effects of training on the decline of VO2max with aging. Federal Proceedings. 46:1830-1833; 1987.
122. Hagberg, J.M.; Graves, J.E.; Limacher, M.; Woods, D.R.; Leggett, S.H.; Cononie, C.; Gruber, J.J.; Pollock, M.L. Cardiovascular responses of 70-79-yr-old men and women to exercise training. Journal of Applied Physiology. 66:2589-2594; 1989.
123. Hakki, A.H.; DePace, N.L.; Iskandrian, A.S. Effect of age on left ventricular function during exercise in patients with coronary artery disease. Journal of the American College of Cardiology. 2:645-651; 1983.
124. Hamm, L.S.; Leon, A.S. Exercise training for the coronary patient. In: Wenger, N.K.; Hellerstein, H.K., eds. Rehabilitation of the coronary patient. 3rd ed. New York: Churchill Livingstone; 1992:367-402.
125. Harkins, S.W.; Chapman, C.R. Detection and decision factors in pain perception in young and elderly men. Pain. 2:253-264; 1976.
126. Harkins, S.W.; Price, D.P.; Martelli, M. The effects of age on pain perception: thermonociception. Journal of Gerontology. 41:58-63; 1986.
127. Harris, R. Clinical geriatric cardiology: management of the elderly patient. Philadelphia: J.B. Lippincott; 1986:197-241.
128. Harrison, T.R.; Dixon, K.; Russell, R.O., Jr.; Bidwai, P.S.; Coleman, H.N. The relation of age to the duration of contraction, ejection, and relaxation of the normal human heart. American Heart Journal. 67:189-199; 1964.
129. Hartzell, A.A.; Freund, B.J.; Jilka, S.M.; Joyner, M.J.; Anderson, R.L.; Ewy, G.A.; Wilmore, J.H. The effects of beta-adrenergic blockade on rating of perceived exertion during submaximal exercise performance following endurance training. Journal of Cardiopulmonary Rehabilitation. 6:444-456; 1986.
130. Hellerstein, H.K.; Hornsten, T.R.; Goldbarg, A.N.; Burlando, A.C.; Friedman, H.; Hirsch, E.Z.; Marik, S. The influence of active conditioning upon subjects with coronary artery disease: a progress report. The Canadian Medical Association Journal. 96:901-903; 1967.
131. Hermanson, B.; Omenn, G.S.; Kronmal, R.A.; Gersh, B.J. Beneficial six-year outcome of smoking cessation in older men and women with coronary artery disease: results from the CASS Registry. New England Journal of Medicine. 319:1365-1369; 1988.
132. Heyward, V.H. Designed for fitness. New York: MacMillan Publishing; 1984:140-150.
133. Horn, J.L.; Donaldson, G. On the myth of intellectual decline in adulthood. The American Psychologist. 31:701-719; 1976.
134. Hulley, S.B.; Furberg, C.D.; Gurland, B.; McDonald, R.; Perry, H.M.; Schnaper, H.W.; Schoenberger, J.A.; Smith, W. McF.; Vogt, T.M. [For the Systolic Hypertension in the Elderly Program (SHEP) research group].

Antihypertensive efficacy of chlorthalidone. American Journal of Cardiology. 56:913-920; 1985.

135. Ike, R.W.; Lampman, R.M.; Castor, C.W. Arthritis and aerobic exercise. Physician and Sportsmedicine. 17(2):128-139; 1989.

136. Imperial, E.S.; Gass, G.; Mitchell, R.; Kelleher, P.; Rayel, R.; Burnker, P.; Baker, P. Graded exercise testing protocol for the elderly. Journal of Cardiopulmonary Rehabilitation. 10:465-470; 1990.

137. Ippolito, E.; Natali, P.G.; Postacchini, F.; Accini, L.; de Martino, C. Morphological, immunochemical, and biochemical study of rabbit achilles tendon at various ages. Journal of Bone and Joint Surgery. 62A:583-598; 1980.

138. Iskandrian, A.S. Single-photon emission computed tomographic thallium imaging with adenosine, dipyridamole, and exercise. American Heart Journal. 122:279-284; 1991.

139. Iskandrian, A.S.; Hakki, A.H. Thallium-201 myocardial scintigraphy. American Heart Journal. 109:113-128; 1985.

140. Iskandrian, A.S.; Heo, J.; Decoskey, D.; Askenase, A.; Segal, B.L. Use of exercise thallium-201 imaging for risk stratification of elderly patients with coronary artery disease. American Journal of Cardiology. 61:269-272; 1988.

141. Jahnigen, D.W. Atrial fibrillation in the elderly: management update. Geriatrics. 45:26-29; 1990.

142. Jajich, C.L.; Ostfeld, A.M.; Freeman, D.H., Jr. Smoking and coronary heart disease mortality in the elderly. Journal of the American Medical Association. 252:2831-2834; 1984.

143. Jamy, P.P. Prescribing for the elderly. Littleton, MA: PSG Publishing; 1980.

144. Julius, S.; Amery, A.; Whitlock, L.S.; Conway, J. Influence of age on a hemodynamic response to exercise. Circulation. 36:222-230; 1967.

145. Kannel, W.B.; Vokonas, P.S. Primary risk factors for coronary heart disease in the elderly: the Framingham study. In: Wenger, N.K.; Furberg, C.D.; Pitt, E., eds. Coronary heart disease in the elderly. New York: Elsevier Science Publishing; 1986:60-92.

146. Kantelip, J.P.; Sage, E.; Duchene-Marullaz, P. Findings on ambulatory electrocardiographic monitoring in subjects older than 80 years. American Journal of Cardiology. 57:398-401; 1986.

147. Kasch, F.W.; Boyer, J.L.; VanCamp, S.P.; Verity, L.S.; Wallace, J.P. The effect of physical activity and inactivity in aerobic power in older men. Physician and Sportsmedicine. 18(4):73-83; 1990.

148. Kasser, I.S.; Bruce, R.A. Comparative effects of aging in coronary heart disease on submaximal and maximal exercise. Circulation. 39:759-774; 1969.

149. Kauffman, T.L. Strength training effect in young and aged women. Archives of Physical Medicine and Rehabilitation. 65:223-226; 1985.

150. Kelemen, M.H.; Stewart, K.J.; Gillilan, R.E.; Ewart, C.K.; Valenti, S.A.; Manley, J.D.; Kellemen, M.D. Circuit weight training in cardiac patients. Journal of the American College of Cardiology. 7:38-42; 1986.

151. Kellerman, J.J.; Ben-Ari, E.; Chayet, M.; Lapidot, C.; Drory, Y.; Fisman, E. Cardio-circulatory response to different types of training in patients with angina pectoris. Cardiology. 62:218-231; 1977.
152. Kennedy, H.L. Comparisons of ambulatory electrocardiography in exercise testing. American Journal of Cardiology. 47:1359-1365; 1981.
153. Kennedy, R.D.; Andrevor, G.R.; Caird, F.I. Ischemic heart disease in the elderly. British Heart Journal. 39:1121-1127; 1977.
154. King, A.C.; Martin, J.E.; Morrell, E.M.; Arena, J.G.; Boland, M.J. Highlighting specific patient education needs in an aging cardiac population. Health Education Quarterly. 13:29-38; 1986.
155. Kiveloff, B.; Huber, O. Brief maximal isometric exercise in hypertension. Journal of the American Geriatric Society. 19:1006-1012; 1971.
156. Kligfield, P.; Ameisen, O.; Okin, P.M. Heart rate adjustment of ST segment depression for improved detection of coronary artery disease. Circulation. 79:245-255; 1989.
157. Lakatta, E.G. Alterations in the cardiovascular system that occur in advanced age. Federation Proceedings. 38:163-167; 1979.
158. Lam, J.Y.G.; Chaitman, B.R.; Glaenzer, M.; Byers, S.; Fite, J.; Shah, Y.; Goodgold, H.; Samuels, L. Safety and diagnostic accuracy of dipyridamole: thallium imaging in the elderly. Journal of the American College of Cardiology. 11:585-589; 1988.
159. Lampman, R.M. Evaluating and prescribing exercise for elderly patients. Geriatrics. 42:63-76; 1987.
160. Larsson, L. Physical training effects on muscle morphology in sedentary males at different ages. Medicine and Science in Sports and Exercise. 14:203-206; 1982.
161. Laslett, L.J.; Amsterdam, E.A.; Mason, D.T. Exercise testing in the geriatric patient. Annals of Internal Medicine. 1:53-61; 1980.
162. Lester, M.; Sheffield, L.T.; Trammell, P.; Reeves, T.J. The effect of age and athletic training on the maximal heart rate during muscular exercise. American Heart Journal. 76:370-376; 1968.
163. Lewis, S.F.; Snell, P.G.; Taylor, W.F.; Hamra, M.; Graham, R.M.; Pettinger, W.A.; Blomqvist, C.G. Role of muscle mass and mode of contraction in circulatory response to exercise. Journal of Applied Physiology. 58:146-151; 1985.
164. Lichtman, S.; Poser, E.G. The effects of exercise on mood and cognitive functioning. The Journal of Psychomotor Research. 27:43-52; 1983.
165. Liemohn, W.P. Strength in aging: an exploratory study. International Journal of Aging and Human Development. 6:347-357; 1975.
166. Lind, A.R.; McNichol, G.W. Muscular forces which determine the cardiovascular responses to sustained and rhythmic exercise. Canadian Medical Association Journal. 96:706-713; 1967.
167. Lowenthal, D.T.; Stein, D.; Hare, T.W.; Yarnoff, A.; Lowenthal, P.J.; Saris, S.; Falkner, B.; Affrime, M.B. The clinical pharmacology of cardiovascular

drugs during exercise. Journal of Cardiopulmonary Rehabilitation. 3:829-837; 1983.

168. Lowenthal, D.T.; Wheat, M.; Kuffler, L.A. Coordinating drug use in exercise and elderly hypertensives. Geriatrics. 43:69-80; 1988.

169. Lund-Johansen, P. Age, hemodynamics, and exercise in essential hypertension: difference between beta blockers and dihydropyridine calcium antagonists. Journal of Cardiovascular Pharmacology. [Suppl. 10]. 14:S7-S13; 1989.

170. Marston, M. Compliance with medical regimens: a review of the literature. Nursing Research. 19:312-323; 1970.

171. Mathes, P. Physical training in patients with ventricular dysfunction: choice and dosage of physical exercise in patients with pump dysfunction. European Heart Journal. [Suppl. F]. 9:67-69; 1988.

172. Mehta, J.; Feldman, R.L.; Marx, J.D.; Kelly, G.A. Systemic, pulmonary, and coronary hemodynamic effects of labetalol in hypertensive subject. American Journal of Medicine. [Suppl. 4A]. 75:32-39; 1983.

173. Miller, P.F.; Sheps, D.S; Bragdon, E.E.; Herbst, M.C.; Dalton, J.L.; Hinderliter, A.L.; Koch, G.G.; Maixner, W.; Ekelund, L.G. Aging and pain perception in ischemic heart disease. American Heart Journal. 120:22-30; 1990.

174. Minor, M.A.; Hewett, J.E.; Webel, R.R.; Anderson, S.K.; Kay, D.R. Efficacy of physical conditioning exercise in patients with rheumatoid arthritis and osteoarthritis. Arthritis and Rheumatism. 32:1396-1405; 1989.

175. Mitman, C.; Edelman, N.H.; Norris, A.H.; Shock, N.W. Relationship between chest wall and pulmonary compliance and age. Journal of Applied Physiology. 70:1211-1216; 1965.

176. Miyatake, K.; Okamoto, J.; Kimoshita, N.; Fusejima, K.; Sakakibara, H.; Nimura, Y. Augmentation of atrial contribution to left ventricular flow with aging as assessed by intra-cardiac doppler flowmetry. American Journal of Cardiology. 53:587-589; 1984.

177. Molloy, D.W.; Beerschoten, D.A.; Borrie, M.J.; Crilly, R.G.; Cape, R.D.T. Acute effects of exercise on neuropsychological function in elderly subjects. Journal of the American Geriatric Society. 36:29-31; 1988.

178. Montgomery, D.L.; Ismail, A.H. The effect of a four-month physical fitness program on high-and-low fit groups matched for age. Journal of Sports Medicine. 17:327-333; 1977.

179. Morgan, W.P.; Roberts, J.A.; Brand, F.R.; Feinerman, A.D. Psychological effect of chronic physical activity. Medicine and Science in Sports. 2:213-217; 1970.

180. Moritani, T.; deVries, H.A. Potential for gross muscle hypertrophy in older men. Journal of Gerontology. 35:672-682; 1980.

181. Nair, C.K.; Sketch, M.H.; Ahmed, I.; Thomson, W.; Ryschon, K.; Woodruff, M.P.; Runco, V. Calcific valvular aortic stenosis with and without mitral annular calcium. American Journal of Cardiology. 60:865-870; 1987.

182. Nair, C.K.; Stading, J. Hypertension in the elderly. Cardiovascular Review and Reports. 13:9-10; 1992.

183. Nair, C.K.; Thomson, W.; Ryschon, K.; Cook, C.; Hee, T.T.; Sketch, M.H. Long-term follow-up of patients with echocardiographically detected mitral annular calcium in comparison with age and sex matched control subjects. American Journal of Cardiology. 63:465-470; 1989.

184. National Center for Health Statistics. 1986 Summary: national hospital discharge survey. Advance data from vital and health services statistics. Available from: United States Public Health Service, Hyattsville, MD: DHHS Publication No. 145 [PHS]. 6:87-1250; 1987.

185. National Cholesterol Education Program Expert Panel. Report of the National Cholesterol Education Program Expert Panel on detection, evaluation, and treatment of high blood cholesterol in adults. Archives of Internal Medicine. 148:36-69; 1988.

186. Naughton, J. Stress electrocardiography and clinical electrocardiographic correlations. Cardiovascular Clinics. 8:127-139; 1977.

187. Ninimaa, V.; Shephard, R.J. Training and oxygen conductance in the elderly: I. The repiratory system. Journal of Gerontology. 33:354-361; 1978.

188. Ninimaa, Z.; Shephard, R.J. Training and oxygen conductance in the elderly. II. The cardiovascular system. Journal of Gerontology. 33:362-367; 1978.

189. Novak, L.P. Aging, total body potassium, fat free mass, and cell mass in males and females between ages 18 and 85 years. Journal of Gerontology. 27:438-443; 1972.

190. Oldridge, N.B. Compliance and drop-out in cardiac exercise rehabilitation. Journal of Cardiac Rehabilitation. 4:166-177; 1984.

191. Oldridge, N.B.; Guyatt, G.H.; Fischer, M.S.; Rimm, A.A. Cardiac rehabilitation after myocardial infarction: combined experience of randomized clinical trials. Journal of the American Medical Association. 260:945-950; 1988.

192. Oldridge, N.B.; LaSalle, D.; Jones, N.L. Exercise rehabilitation of female patients with coronary artery disease. American Heart Journal. 100:755-757; 1980.

193. Opie, L.H.; Sonnenblick, E.H.; Kaplan, N.M.; Thadani, U. Beta-blocking agents. In: Opie, L.H., ed. Drugs for the heart. 3rd ed. Philadelphia: W.B. Saunders; 1991;1-25.

194. O'Rourke, R.A.; Chatterjee, K.; Wei, J.Y. Coronary heart disease. 18th Bethesda conference report: cardiovascular disease in the elderly. Journal of the American College of Cardiology. 10:52A-56A; 1987.

195. Packard, B. Clinical aspects of coronary heart disease in women. In: Wenger, N.K.; Hellerstein, H.K., eds. Rehabilitation of the coronary patient. 3rd ed. New York: Churchill Livingstone; 1992:217-230.

196. Pashkow, F.J. Patients with implanted pacemakers or implanted cardioverter defibrillators. In: Wenger, N.K.; Hellerstein, H.K., eds. Rehabilitation of the coronary patient. 2nd ed. New York: Churchill Livingstone; 1992:431-438.

197. Perkins, L.C.; Kaiser, H.L. Results of short-term isotonic and isometric exercise programs in persons over 60. Physical Therapy Review. 41:633-635; 1961.

198. Petratis, M.M.; Williams, M.A.; Fogland, T.L.; Esterbrooks, D.J. The benefits of early exercise training in female cardiac patients. Journal of Cardiac Rehabilitation. [Abstract]. 7:503; 1987.

199. Pfeiffer, E. Psychopathology and social pathology. In: Birren, J.E.; Schaie, K.W., eds. Handbook of the psychology of aging. New York: Van Nostrand Reinhold; 1977:650-671.

200. Pollock, M.L.; Ward, A.; Foster, C. Exercise prescription for rehabilitation of the cardiac patient. In: Pollock, M.L.; Schmidt, D.H., eds. Heart disease and rehabilitation. Boston: Houghton Mifflin; 1979:413-445.

201. Pollock, M.L.; Wilmore, J.H. Exercise in health and disease. Evaluation and prescription for prevention and rehabilitation. 2nd ed. Philadelphia: W.B. Saunders; 1990.

202. Posner, J.D.; Gorman, K.M.; Klein, H.S.; Woldow, A. Exercise capacity in the elderly. American Journal of Cardiology. 57:52C-58C; 1986.

203. Post, F. Dementia, depression, and pseudo-dementia. In: Benson, D.F.; Blumer, D., eds. Psychiatric aspects of neurological disease. New York: Grune & Stratton; 1975:99-120.

204. Powell, R.R. Psychological effects of exercise therapy upon institutionalized geriatric mental patients. Journal of Gerontology. 29:157-161; 1974.

205. Preventive and Rehabilitative Exercise Committee, American College of Sports Medicine. Guidelines for exercise testing and prescription. 4th ed. Philadelphia: Lea & Febiger, 1991.

206. Reaven, G.M. Role of insulin resistance in human disease. Diabetes. 37:1595-1607; 1988.

207. Rich, M.W.; Palmeri, S.; McCluskey, E.R.; Schwartz, J.B. Calcium channel blockers for hypertension in older patients. Cardiovascular Review and Reports. 12:11-14; 1991.

208. Rodahl, K. The effects of physical conditioning on older individuals: I. Work capacity, circulatory-respiratory function, and work electrocardiogram. Journal of Gerontology. 21:182-191; 1966.

209. Rodeheffer, R.J.; Gerstenblith, G.; Becker, L.C.; Fleg, J.L.; Weisfeldt, M.L.; Lakatta, E.G. Exercise cardiac output is maintained with advancing age in healthy human subjects: cardiac dilatation and increased stroke volume compensate for a diminished heart rate. Circulation. 69:203-213; 1984.

210. Rosenthal, M.; Doberne, L.; Greenfield, M.; Widstrom, A.; Reaven, G.M. Effect of age on glucose tolerance, insulin secretion, and in vivo insulin action. Journal of the Geriatric Society. 30:562-567; 1982.

211. Rubin, S.M.; Sidney, S.; Black, D.M.; Browner, W.S.; Hulley, S.B.; Cummings, S.R. High cholesterol in elderly men and the excess risk for coronary heart disease. Annals of Internal Medicine. 113:916-920; 1990.

212. Saltin, B. The aging endurance athlete. In: Sutton, J.R.; Brock, R., eds. Sports medicine for the mature athlete. Indianapolis: Benchmark Press; 1986:59-80.

213. Saltin, B.; Lingarde, F.; Houston, M.; Horlin, R.; Nugaard, E.; Gad, P. Physical training and glucose tolerance in middle-aged men with chemical diabetes. Diabetes. 28:30-32; 1979.

214. Satler, L.F.; Green, C.E.; Wallace, R.B.; Rackley, C.E. Coronary artery disease in the elderly. American Journal of Cardiology. 63:245-248; 1989.

215. Saunamaki, K.I. Early post-myocardial infarction exercise testing in subjects 70 years or more of age: functional and prognostic evaluation. European Heart Journal. [Suppl. E]. 5:93-96; 1984.

216. Savin, W.M.; Haskell, W.L.; Houston-Miller, N.; DeBusk, R. Improvement in aerobic capacity soon after myocardial infarction. Journal of Cardiac Rehabilitation. 1:337-342; 1981.

217. Schang, S.J.; Pepine, C.J. Transient asymptomatic ST segment depression during daily activity.

218. Schrager, B.R.; Ellestad, M.H. The importance of blood pressure measurement during exercise testing. Cardiovascular Review and Reports. 4:381-394; 1983.

219. Seals, D.R.; Hagberg, J.M.; Hurley, B.F.; Ehsani, A.A.; Holloszy, J.O. Endurance training in older men and women: I. Cardiovascular responses to exercise. Journal of Applied Physiology. 57:1024-1029; 1984.

220. Seals, D.R.; Hurley, B.F.; Schultz, J.; Hagberg, J.M. Endurance training in older men and women: II. Blood lactate responses to submaximal exercise. Journal of Applied Physiology. 57:1030-1031; 1984.

221. Sheffield, C.T. Graded exercise test (GXT) for ischemic heart disease: a submaximal test to a target heart rate. In: Exercise testing and training of apparently healthy individuals: a handbook for physicians. Dallas: American Heart Association; 1972:35-38.

222. Shephard, R.J. Physical training for the elderly. Clinics In Sports Medicine. 5:515-533; 1986.

223. Shephard, R.J. Physical activity and aging. 2nd ed. Rockville, MD: Aspen Publishers; 1987.

224. Shephard, R.J. Prescribing exercise for the senior citizen: some simple guidelines. Chicago: Chicago Yearbook; 1989.

225. Sheps, D.S. Exercise-induced diastolic increase: indicator of severe coronary disease. Primary Cardiology Clinics. 4:14-21; 1980.

226. Shock, N.W. Physiological aspects of aging in man. Annual Review of Physiology. 23:97-122; 1961.

227. Sidney, K.H.; Shephard, R.J. Attitudes towards health and physical activity in the elderly. Medicine and Science in Sports. 8:246-252; 1976.

228. Sidney, K.H.; Shephard, R.J. Maximum and submaximum exercise tests in men and women in seventh, eighth, and ninth decades of life. Journal of Applied Physiology. 43:280-287; 1977.

229. Sidney, K.H.; Shephard, R.J. Training and electrocardiographic abnormalities in the elderly. British Heart Journal. 39:1114-1120; 1977.

230. Sidney, K.H.; Shephard, R.J. Frequency and intensity of exercise training for elderly subjects. Medicine and Science in Sports. 10:125-131; 1978.

231. Sidney, K.H.; Shephard, R.J.; Harrison, J. Endurance training and body composition of the elderly. American Journal of Clinical Nutrition. 30:326-333; 1977.

232. Siegel, D.; Kuller, L.; Lazarus, N.B.; Black, D.; Feigal, D.; Hughes, G.; Schoenberger, J.A.; Hulley, S.B. Predictors of cardiovascular events and mortality in the Systolic Hypertension in the Elderly Program Pilot Project. American Journal of Epidemiology. 126:385-399; 1987.

233. Siffring, P.A.; Gupta, N.C.; Mohiuddin, S.M.; Esterbrooks, D.J.; Hilleman, D.E.; Cheng, S.C.; Sketch, M.H., Sr.; Frick, M.P. Myocardial uptake and clearance of thallium-201 in healthy subjects: comparison of adenosine-induced hyperemia and exercise stress. Radiology. 173:769-774; 1989.

234. Simons, C.W.; Birkimer, J.C. An exploration of factors predicting the effects of aerobic conditioning on mood state. The Journal of Psychomotor Research. 32:63-85; 1988.

235. Simonson, E. The effect of age on the electrocardiogram. American Journal of Cardiology. 29:64-73; 1972.

236. Sjogren, A.L. Left ventricular wall thickness in patients with circulatory overload of the left ventricle. Clinical Research. 4:310-318; 1972.

237. Sketch, M.H.; Mooss, A.N.; Butler, M.L.; Nair, C.K.; Mohiuddin, S.M. Digoxin-induced positive exercise tests: their clinical and prognostic significance. American Journal of Cardiology. 48:655-659; 1981.

238. Smith, D.M.; Khairi, M.R.; Norton, J. Age and activity effects on rate of bone mineral loss. Journal of Clinical Investigation. 58:716-721; 1976.

239. Smith, E.L.; Gilligan, C. Physical activity prescription for the older adult. Physician and Sportsmedicine. 11(8):91-101; 1983.

240. Smith, E.L.; Serfass, R.C. Exercise and aging: the scientific basis. Hillside, NJ: Enslow Publishers; 1981.

241. Snowdon, D.A.; Phillips, P.L.; Fraser, G.E. Meat consumption and fatal ischemic heart disease. Preventive Medicine. 13:490-500; 1984.

242. Sparrow, D.; Dawber, T.R.; Colton, T. The influence of cigarette smoking on prognosis after a first myocardial infarction. Journal of Chronic Diseases. 31:425-432; 1978.

243. Spirduso, W.W. Physical fitness, aging, and psychomotor speed: a review. Journal of Gerontology. 35:850-865; 1980.

244. Stamford, B.A. Physiologic effects of training upon institutionalized geriatric men. Journal of Gerontology. 27:451-455; 1972.

245. Stamford, B.A.; Hambacher, W.; Fallica, A. Effects of daily exercise on the psychiatric state of institutionalized geriatric mental patients. Research Quarterly. 45:34-41; 1974.

246. Stout, R.W. Overview of the association between insulin and atherosclerosis. Metabolism. [Suppl. 1]. 34:7-12; 1985.

247. Strasser, T. Cardiovascular care of the elderly. Geneva, Switzerland: World Health Organization; 1987:79-90.

248. Stratmann, H.G.; Kennedy, H.L. Evaluation of coronary artery disease in the patient unable to exercise: alternatives to exercise stress testing. American Heart Journal. 117:1344-1365; 1989.

249. Subcommittee on Rehabilitation Target Activity Group, American Heart Association. Standards for adult exercise testing laboratories. Circulation. 59:421A-427A; 1979.

250. Sullivan, M.J.; Knight, J.D.; Higginbotham, M.B.; Cobb, F.R. Relation between central and peripheral hemodynamics during exercise in patients with chronic heart failure: also blood flow is reduced with maintenance or arterial perfusion pressure. Circulation. 80:769-781; 1989.

251. Thomas, S.G.; Cunningham, D.A.; Rechnitzer, P.A.; Donner, A.P.; Howard, J.H. Determinants of the training response in elderly men. Medicine and Science in Sports and Exercise. 17:667-672; 1985.

252. Thompson, R.F.; Crist, D.M.; Marsh, M.; Rosenthal, M. Effects of physical exercise for elderly patients with physical impairments. Journal of the American Geriatric Society. 36:130-135; 1988.

253. Tinetti, M.E.; Speechley, M.; Ginter, S.F. Risk factors for falls among elderly persons living in the community. New England Journal of Medicine. 319:1701-1707; 1988.

254. Vander, L.B.; Franklin, B.A.; Wrisley, D.; Rubenfire, M. Acute cardiovascular responses to Nautilus exercise in cardiac patients: implications for exercise training. Annals of Sports Medicine. 2:165-169; 1986.

255. Vasilomanolakis, E.C. Geriatric cardiology: when exercise stress testing is justified. Journal of Geriatrics. 40:47-57; 1985.

256. Vasilomanolakis, E.C.; Damian, A.; Mahan, G.; Baron, D.; Ellestad, M. Treadmill stress testing in geriatric patients. Journal of the American College of Cardiology. [Abstract]. 3:520; 1984.

257. Verani, M.S. Adenosine thallium-201 myocardial perfusion scintigraphy. American Heart Journal. 122:269-278; 1991.

258. Verani, M.S.; Mahmarian, J.J.; Hixson, J.B.; Boyce, T.M.; Staudacher, R.A. Diagnosis of coronary artery disease by controlled coronary vasodilatation with adenosine and thallium-201 scintigraphy in patients unable to exercise. Circulation. 82:80-87; 1990.

259. Wasserman, K. The peripheral circulation and lactic acid metabolism in heart or cardiovascular failure. Circulation. 80:1084-1086; 1989.

260. Wayne, V.S.; Fagan, E.T.; McConachy, D.L. The effects of isosorbide dinitrate on the exercise test. Journal of Cardiopulmonary Rehabilitation. 7:239-252; 1987.

261. Wear, C.L. The relationship of flexibility measurements to length of body segments. Research Quarterly. 34:234-238; 1963.

262. Weiner, D.A.; Ryan, T.J.; Parsons, L.; Fisher, L.D.; Chaitman, B.R.; Sheffield, L.T.; Tristiani, F.E. Significance of silent myocardial ischemia during exercise testing in patients with diabetes mellitus: a report from the Coronary Artery Surgery Study (CASS) Registry. American Journal of Cardiology. 68:729-734; 1991.

263. Weingarten, G.; Alexander, J.F. The effects of physical exertion on mental performance of college males of different physical fitness levels. Perceptual Motor Skills. 31:371-378; 1970.

264. Wenger, N.K. The elderly coronary patient. In: Wenger, N.K.; Hellerstein, H.K., eds. Rehabilitation of the coronary patient. 2nd ed. New York: John Wiley & Sons; 1984:397-409.

265. Wenger, N.K. Coronary heart disease. 18th Bethesda conference report: cardiovascular disease in the elderly. Journal of the American College of Cardiology. 10:8A-9A; 1987.

266. Wenger, N.K. Coronary heart disease in the elderly. In: Wenger, N.K.; Hellerstein, H.K., eds. Rehabilitation of the coronary patient. 3rd ed. New York: Churchill Livingstone; 1992:211-215.

267. Wenger, N.K. Patients with left ventricular dysfunction and congestive heart failure. In: Wenger, N.K.; Hellerstein, H.K., eds. Rehabilitation of the coronary patient. 3rd ed. New York: Churchill Livingstone; 1992:403-413.

268. Wenger, N.K. Rehabilitation of the coronary patient in the 21st century: challenges and opportunities. In: Wenger, N.K.; Hellerstein, H.K., eds. Rehabilitation of the coronary patient. 3rd ed. New York: Churchill Livingstone; 1992:581-592.

269. White, N.K.; Edwards, J.E.; Dry, T.J. The relationship of the degree of coronary atherosclerosis with age. Circulation. 1:645-654; 1950.

270. Wilhelmsson, L.; Elmfeldt, D.; Vedin, J.A.; Tibblin, G.; Wilhelmsen, L. Smoking and myocardial infarction. Lancet. 1:415-420; 1975.

271. Williams, M.A. Principles and methods of exercise testing. In: Fardy, P.S.; Bennett, J.L.; Reitz, N.L.; Williams, M.A., eds. Cardiac rehabilitation: implications for the nurse and other health professionals. St. Louis: C.V. Mosby; 1980:52-72.

272. Williams, M.A. Prevalence of reduced exercise capacity and coronary risk factors in elderly cardiac patients: implications for rehabilitation programs. Journal of Cardiopulmonary Rehabilitation. [Abstract]. 9:410; 1989.

273. Williams, M.A.; Docken, T.L.; Monnig, M.L.; Hilleman, D.E.; Esterbrooks, D.J.; Gupta, N.C.; Mohiuddin, S.M. The use of dynamic exercise or adenosine thallium in the evaluation of coronary artery disease in elderly females. Journal of Cardiopulmonary Rehabilitation. [Abstract]. 11:307; 1991.

273a. Williams, M.A.; Esterbrooks, D.J. Exercise training in the elderly cardiac patient. In: Tresch, D.D.; Aronow, W.S., eds. Management of cardiovascular disease in the elderly patient. New York: Marcel Dekker; in press.

274. Williams, M.A.; Esterbrooks, D.J.; Aronow, W.S.; Sketch, M.H., Sr. Limitations of exercise testing to screen cardiac patients for early non-monitored rehabilitation exercise programs. Journal of Cardiac Rehabilitation. 4:396-401; 1984.

275. Williams, M.A., Esterbrooks, D.J.; Sketch, M.H. Guidelines to exercise therapy of the elderly after myocardial infarction. European Heart Journal. [Suppl. E]. 5:121-123; 1984.

276. Williams, M.A.; Esterbrooks, D.J.; Sketch, M.H., Sr. Limitations of Phase II exercise training in the "older" elderly cardiac patient. Circulation. [Abstract]. 82:III-576; 1990.

277. Williams, M.A.; Esterbrooks, D.J.; Sketch, M.H., Sr. Extension of Phase II exercise training produces significant benefit in the older elderly participant. Journal of Cardiopulmonary Rehabilitation. [Abstract]. 11:312; 1991.

278. Williams, M.A.; Maresh, C.M.; Esterbrooks, D.J.; Harbrecht, J.J.; Sketch, M.H., Sr. Early exercise training in patients older than age 65 years compared with that in younger patients after acute myocardial infarction or coronary artery bypass grafting. American Journal of Cardiology. 55:263-266; 1985.

279. Williams, M.A.; Maresh, C.M.; Esterbrooks, D.J.; Sketch, M.H., Sr. Characteristics of exercise responses following short and long term aerobic training in elderly cardiac patients. Journal of the American Geriatric Society. [Abstract]. 35:904; 1987.

280. Williams, M.A.; Sketch, M.H. Guidelines for exercise training of elderly patients following myocardial infarction and coronary bypass graft surgery. Geriatric Cardiovascular Medicine. 1:107-110; 1988.

281. Williams, M.A.; Sketch, M.H., Sr. After a heart attack: prescribing exercise to speed recovery. Senior Patient. 2:16-20; 1990.

282. Williams, M.A; Smith, L.K. Exercise training elderly cardiac patients. A colloquium at the American College of Sports Medicine Annual Meeting. Dallas, TX; 1992 May 28.

283. Wong, N.D.; Wilson, P.W.F.; Kannel, W.B. Serum cholesterol as a prognostic factor after myocardial infarction: the Framingham study. Annals of Internal Medicine. 115:687-693; 1991.

284. Zoghbi, W.A. Use of adenosine echocardiography for diagnosis of coronary artery disease. American Heart Journal. 122:285-292; 1991.

Index

About the Author

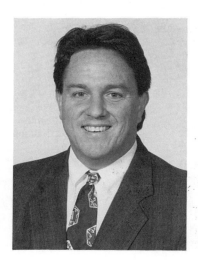

Mark Williams is an associate professor of medicine in the division of cardiology at Creighton University in Omaha, Nebraska, where he has served as the director of the Cardiovascular Disease Prevention and Rehabilitation Program since 1980. Dr. Williams was one of the first to study exercise training in elderly cardiac patients; his paper ''Early Exercise Training in Patients Older Than Age 65 Years Compared With That in Younger Patients After Acute Myocardial Infarction or Coronary Artery Bypass Grafting'' (*American Journal of Cardiology*) was the first research published on this special population.

Dr. Williams is the 1993-1994 president of the American Association of Cardiovascular and Pulmonary Rehabilitation and a fellow of the American College of Sports Medicine. He earned his PhD in exercise physiology and cardiac rehabilitation in 1980 from Texas A & M University.